CONTENTS

BREAKFAST AND BRUNCH

1. Italian Garden Frittata

Servings: 4
Cooking Time: 30 Min
Ingredients:
- 4 large eggs
- 6 large egg whites
- 1/2 cup grated Romano cheese, divided
- 1 tablespoon minced fresh sage
- 1/2 teaspoon salt
- 1/4 teaspoon pepper
- 1 teaspoon olive oil
- 1 small zucchini, sliced
- 2 green onions, sliced
- 2 plum tomatoes, thinly sliced

Directions:
1.   Preheat broiler. In a large bowl, whisk eggs, egg whites, 1/4 cup cheese, sage, salt and pepper until blended.
2.   In a 10-in. broiler-safe skillet coated with cooking spray, heat oil over medium-high heat. Add zucchini and green onions; cook and stir 2 minutes. Reduce heat to medium-low. Pour in egg mixture. Cook, covered, 4-7 minutes or until eggs are nearly set.
3.   Uncover; top with tomatoes and remaining cheese. Broil 3-4 in. from heat 2-3 minutes or until eggs are completely set. Let stand 5 minutes. Cut frittata into wedges.

2. Ham And Avocado Scramble

Servings: 4
Cooking Time: 15 Min
Ingredients:
- 8 large eggs
- 1/4 cup 2% milk
- 1 teaspoon garlic powder
- 1/4 teaspoon pepper
- 1 cup cubed fully cooked ham
- 1 tablespoon butter
- 1 medium ripe avocado, peeled and cubed
- 1 cup (4 ounces) shredded Colby-Monterey Jack cheese

Directions:
1.   In a large bowl, whisk the eggs, milk, garlic powder and pepper; stir in ham. In a large skillet, melt butter over medium-high heat. Add egg mixture; cook and stir until almost set. Stir in avocado and cheese. Cook and stir until completely set.

3. Good Morning Frittata

Servings: 2
Cooking Time: 20 Min
Ingredients:
- 1 cup egg substitute
- 1/4 cup fat-free milk
- 1/8 teaspoon pepper
- Dash salt
- 1/4 cup chopped sweet orange pepper
- 2 green onions, thinly sliced
- 1/2 teaspoon canola oil
- 1/3 cup cubed fully cooked ham
- 1/4 cup shredded reduced-fat cheddar cheese

Directions:

1.   In a small bowl, whisk the egg substitute, milk, pepper and salt; set aside. In an 8-in. ovenproof skillet, saute orange pepper and onions in oil until tender. Add ham; heat through. Reduce heat; top with egg mixture. Cover and cook for 4-6 minutes or until nearly set.

2.   Uncover skillet; sprinkle with cheese. Broil 3-4 in. from the heat for 2-3 minutes or until eggs are completely set. Let stand for 5 minutes. Cut into wedges.

4.   Calico Scrambled Eggs

Servings: 4
Cooking Time: 20 Min
Ingredients:

- 8 large eggs
- 1/4 cup 2% milk
- 1/8 to 1/4 teaspoon dill weed
- 1/8 to 1/4 teaspoon salt
- 1/8 to 1/4 teaspoon pepper
- 1 tablespoon butter
- 1/2 cup chopped green pepper
- 1/4 cup chopped onion
- 1/2 cup chopped fresh tomato

Directions:

1.   In a large bowl, whisk the first five ingredients until blended. In a 12-in. nonstick skillet, heat butter over medium-high heat. Add the green pepper and onion; cook and stir until tender. Remove from pan.

2.   In same pan, pour in egg mixture; cook and stir over medium heat until eggs begin to thicken. Add tomato and pepper mixture; cook until heated through and no liquid egg remains, stirring gently.

5.   Mediterranean Frittata

Servings: 2
Cooking Time: 12 Minutes
Ingredients:

- 3 eggs
- ¼ cup feta cheese, crumbled
- 2 tbsps. pitted kalamata olives
- ¼ tsp oregano
- ½ cup milk
- Salt and pepper to taste
- 2 cherry tomatoes halved
- 1 ½ tbsps. olive oil

Directions:

1.   Crack the eggs and beat with milk in a bowl. Season with the oregano, salt, and pepper.

2.   Grease the iron skillet and heat on medium heat.

3.   Add the egg mixture. Fold the edges of the frittata with a spatula and cook the eggs halfway through.

4.   Add the crumbled feta cheese and sliced tomatoes on top and pop the skillet in the oven. Cook at 380F for 5 to 6 minutes.

5.   Cool, slice, and serve.

6.   Fried Bologna And Egg Sandwich

Servings: 2
Cooking Time: 15 Minutes
Ingredients:

- 2 slices bologna
- 1 tablespoon salted butter
- 2 large eggs

- Pinch sea salt
- 4 slices bread
- 1 tablespoon mayonnaise

Directions:

1. Heat the skillet over medium heat. Place the bologna in the hot skillet and cook for 2 to 3 minutes per side, until well browned. Transfer the bologna to a plate and loosely cover it with a clean kitchen towel to keep it warm. Set aside.
2. Still at medium heat, melt the butter in the skillet. Crack the eggs into the skillet so they are evenly spaced. Sprinkle salt over the yolks. For over-easy eggs, cook for about 4 minutes, until the whites have cooked through (about 5 minutes for over-medium, and about 6 minutes for over-well), flip the eggs while the yolks are still liquid, being careful not to break them. Cook for 1 minute more and remove from the heat.
3. While the eggs cook, toast the bread.
4. Spread the mayonnaise evenly on each slice of bread and assemble each sandwich with 1 egg and 1 piece of bologna.

7. Caramelized Cream-fried Eggs Over Parmesan Grits

Servings: 2
Cooking Time: 20 Minutes
Ingredients:

- 1 cup stone-ground grits
- 3 cups water
- 1½ cups heavy (whipping) cream, divided
- 1 tablespoon sea salt, plus ½ teaspoon
- 1 tablespoon salted butter
- ½ cup grated Parmesan cheese
- 4 large eggs

Directions:

1. In a medium saucepan over high heat, stir together the grits, water, 1 cup of cream, and 1 tablespoon of salt until well combined. Bring to a boil. Reduce the heat to low, cover the saucepan, and simmer for about 20 minutes, until the grits have thickened. Stir in the butter and Parmesan cheese.
2. Once the grits have cooked for 10 minutes, pour the remaining ½ cup of cream into the skillet. Crack the eggs into the cream and season them with the remaining ½ teaspoon of salt.
3. Place the skillet over medium-high heat and cook for 6 to 7 minutes, or until the whites have set and the cream has begun to brown (the eggs will cook as the cream caramelizes). Remove the skillet from the heat, cover it, and let sit for 1 to 2 minutes to let the whites firm up.
4. Divide the grits into 2 serving bowls. Top each serving with 2 eggs and a spoonful of cream and serve.

8. Tortilla Española

Servings: 6 To 8
Cooking Time: 35 To 40 Minutes
Ingredients:

- 2 cups olive oil
- 2 Yukon Gold potatoes, peeled and thinly sliced
- 1 large white onion
- 8 large eggs
- Pinch sea salt

Directions:

1. Heat the oil in your skillet over medium-low heat.
2. Add the potatoes and onions to the skillet and simmer until tender, 20 to 25 minutes.
3. Strain the potatoes and onions into a bowl and drain off the oil, setting aside 2 tablespoons.
4. Whisk the eggs in a large bowl until frothing. Stir the potatoes and onions into the eggs, along with the salt.
5. Return 1 tablespoon of olive oil to the pan and heat over medium heat. When the oil is hot, pour the egg and potato mixture into the pan, cooking for 7 to 10 minutes. When the eggs have set and the bottom has started to brown, remove the pan from the heat.

6. Place a plate—large enough to cover the entire skillet—on top and flip the tortilla out of the pan. Return the pan to the heat, adding the remaining olive oil, and slide the tortilla back into the pan, golden-side up. Cook for an additional 5 minutes, until both sides are golden brown. Flip once more onto a plate, slice, and serve.

9. Hash Brown & Apple Pancake

Servings: 4
Cooking Time: 20 Min
Ingredients:
- 1 1/4 cups frozen shredded hash brown potatoes, thawed
- 1/2 cup finely chopped apple
- 1/4 cup finely chopped onion
- 1 large egg white
- 1 tablespoon minced fresh chives
- 1/4 teaspoon salt
- 1/4 teaspoon pepper
- 2 tablespoons butter, divided
- 2 tablespoons canola oil, divided
- 1/2 cup shredded Swiss cheese

Directions:
1. In a large bowl, combine the first seven ingredients. In a large nonstick skillet, heat 1 tablespoon butter and 1 tablespoon oil over medium-high heat.
2. Spread half of the potato mixture evenly in pan; sprinkle with cheese. Top with remaining potato mixture, pressing gently into skillet. Cook 5 minutes or until bottom is browned.
3. Carefully invert pancake onto a plate. Heat remaining butter and oil in same pan. Slide pancake into skillet, browned side up. Cook 5 minutes longer or until bottom is browned and cheese is melted. Slide pancake onto a plate; cut into four wedges.

10. Breakfast Sausage Patties

Servings: 2
Cooking Time: 10 Minutes
Ingredients:
- ½ pound ground pork
- ½ tbsp fresh sage leaves, chopped
- ½ tsp brown sugar
- ¼ tsp freshly ground nutmeg
- ½ tsp salt
- 2 tsp cayenne pepper
- Pepper to taste
- Oil for cooking

Directions:
1. Combine everything (except for the oil) in a bowl and mix with your hands.
2. Make 4 patties.
3. Grease the skillet with oil and cook the patties for 4 to 5 minutes per side.
4. Serve.

11. Fried Grits With Strawberries And Honey

Servings: 4 To 6
Cooking Time: 40 Minutes
Ingredients:
- ½ cup stone-ground grits
- 1 cup water
- 1 cup whole milk
- 1 tablespoon honey

- Pinch sea salt
- 1 teaspoon ground cinnamon
- 4 tablespoons salted butter
- ½ cup all-purpose flour
- FOR THE TOPPING
- 1 pint fresh strawberries, hulled and sliced
- 3 tablespoons honey
- 2 tablespoons powdered sugar

Directions:
1. In a medium saucepan combine the grits, water, milk, honey, salt, and cinnamon. Bring to a boil and then reduce the heat to a simmer. Cook for about 20 minutes, stirring frequently, until the grits are thick but still creamy.
2. Using a small amount of the butter, grease a 9 x 9" baking dish and pour the grit mixture into the pan. Chill for at least 1 hour, preferably overnight.
3. Combine the strawberries and honey for the topping and set aside.
4. Melt 1 tablespoon of butter in your skillet over medium heat.
5. Slice the grits into 3" squares. Use a spoon to coat the top and bottom of the squares with flour.
6. Transfer 4 squares to the hot skillet and fry for 2 to 3 minutes per side, until crispy.
7. As the grits squares come off the skillet, keep them warm in the microwave or in a 200°F oven on a baking sheet.
8. Fry the remaining squares, adding butter to the pan between each batch.
9. Serve hot, topped with the fresh berries and honey and a sprinkle of powdered sugar.

12. Triple-berry Breakfast Clafoutis With Almonds

Servings: 2
Cooking Time: 50 Minutes
Ingredients:
- 2/3 tbsp. unsalted butter, melted, plus more at room temperature for greasing
- ¼ cup of sugar
- 2 tbsps. all-purpose flour
- 1 egg
- ½ cup whole milk
- ½ tsp. vanilla extract
- A pinch of salt
- 1/3 cup fresh blueberries
- 1/3 cup fresh raspberries
- 1/3 cup fresh, quartered strawberries
- 2 tbsps. sliced almonds

Directions:
1. Preheat the oven to 350F. Grease a cast iron with butter.
2. Blend the melted butter, sugar, flour, eggs, milk, vanilla, and salt in a blender.
3. Pour the batter into the skillet and scatter the berries over the batter. Then scatter the almonds.
4. Bake for 35 to 45 minutes, or until a tester inserted in the middle comes out clean.
5. Slice and serve.

13. Spanish Omelet

Servings: 2
Cooking Time: 15 Min
Ingredients:
- 6 large eggs
- 1/4 cup water
- 1 cup refried beans, warmed
- 1/4 cup chopped red onion
- 1/2 cup shredded Mexican cheese blend, divided
- 1/4 cup salsa

Directions:
1. Heat a 10-in. nonstick skillet coated with cooking spray over medium heat. Whisk eggs and water. Add half of the egg mixture to skillet (mixture should set immediately at edges).
2. As the eggs set, push the cooked edges toward the center, letting the uncooked portion flow underneath. When the eggs are set, spoon half of the beans and half of the onion on one side and sprinkle with 2 tablespoons cheese; fold other side over filling. Slide omelet onto a plate. Repeat. Garnish with salsa and remaining cheese.

14. Roasted Red Pepper And Goat Cheese Frittata

Servings: 6
Cooking Time: 55 Minutes
Ingredients:
- 2 red bell peppers, halved and seeded
- 1 tablespoon olive oil
- 2 tablespoons salted butter
- 1 white onion, chopped
- 2 garlic cloves, minced
- 6 large eggs
- ¼ cup heavy (whipping) cream
- ½ teaspoon sea salt
- 1 cup goat cheese, crumbled

Directions:
1. Preheat the oven to 400°F.
2. Place the pepper halves into the skillet and drizzle them with oil. Roast for 20 minutes, until the peppers begin to brown. Flip the peppers and roast for 10 minutes more, then remove them from the oven. Keep the oven at 400°F. Roughly chop the peppers and set aside.
3. In the skillet over medium heat, melt the butter. Add the onion and cook for 5 to 7 minutes, stirring occasionally, until softened. Add the garlic and cook for 2 minutes, or until fragrant.
4. Meanwhile, in a large bowl, whisk the eggs, cream, and salt to blend. Stir in the roasted red peppers and goat cheese. Pour the mixture into the skillet and cook for 1 to 2 minutes, or until the eggs just begin to set.
5. Transfer the skillet to the oven. Bake for 10 to 12 minutes, or until the frittata is cooked through.

15. Ham Steaks With Gruyere, Bacon & Mushrooms

Servings: 4
Cooking Time: 25 Min
Ingredients:
- 2 tablespoons butter
- 1/2 pound sliced fresh mushrooms
- 1 shallot, finely chopped
- 2 garlic cloves, minced
- 1/8 teaspoon coarsely ground pepper
- 1 fully cooked boneless ham steak (about 1 pound), cut into four pieces
- 1 cup (4 ounces) shredded Gruyere cheese
- 4 bacon strips, cooked and crumbled
- 1 tablespoon minced fresh parsley, optional

Directions:
1. In a large nonstick skillet, heat butter over medium-high heat. Add mushrooms and shallot; cook and stir 4-6 minutes or until tender. Add garlic and pepper; cook 1 minute longer. Remove from pan; keep warm. Wipe skillet clean.
2. In same skillet, cook ham over medium heat 3 minutes. Turn; sprinkle with cheese and bacon. Cook, covered, 2-4 minutes longer or until cheese is melted and ham is heated through. Serve with mushroom mixture. If desired, sprinkle with parsley.

16. French Banana Pancakes

Servings: 5-6
Cooking Time: 30 Min
Ingredients:
- PANCAKES
- 1 cup all-purpose flour
- 1/4 cup confectioners' sugar
- 1 cup milk
- 2 large eggs
- 3 tablespoons butter, melted
- 1 teaspoon vanilla extract
- 1/4 teaspoon salt
- FILLING
- 1/4 cup butter
- 1/4 cup packed brown sugar
- 1/4 teaspoon ground cinnamon
- 1/4 teaspoon ground nutmeg
- 1/4 cup half-and-half cream
- 5 to 6 firm bananas, halved lengthwise
- Whipped cream and additional cinnamon, optional

Directions:
1. Sift flour and confectioners' sugar into a bowl. Add milk, eggs, butter, vanilla and salt; beat until smooth.
2. Heat a lightly greased 6-in. skillet; add about 3 tablespoons batter, spreading to almost cover bottom of skillet. Cook until lightly browned; turn and brown the other side. Remove to a wire rack. Repeat with remaining batter (make 10-12 pancakes), greasing skillet as needed.
3. For filling, melt butter in large skillet. Stir in brown sugar, cinnamon and nutmeg. Stir in cream and cook until slightly thickened. Add half of the bananas at a time to skillet; heat for 2-3 minutes, spooning sauce over them. Remove from the heat.
4. Roll a pancake around each banana half and place on a serving platter. Spoon sauce over pancakes. Top with whipped cream and dash of cinnamon if desired.

17. Blackberry And White Chocolate Dutch Baby

Servings: 2 To 4
Cooking Time: 20 Minutes
Ingredients:
- 1 cup buttermilk
- 3 eggs
- 2 tablespoons packed brown sugar
- 1 teaspoon vanilla extract
- Pinch sea salt
- ¾ cup all-purpose flour
- 5 tablespoons salted butter
- 1 cup fresh blackberries
- 2 tablespoons honey
- ½ cup white chocolate chips
- Maple syrup, for serving

Directions:
1. Adjust your oven rack to the middle position, place your empty skillet on it, and preheat the oven to 425°F.
2. In a medium bowl, whisk together the buttermilk, eggs, brown sugar, vanilla, and salt.
3. Fold in the flour gently until blended. Let the batter rest for 5 minutes.
4. Remove the hot skillet from the oven, add the butter, and let it melt.
5. Pour the batter into the skillet and immediately return it to the oven. Bake for 15 to 20 minutes or until the pancake is golden brown and the sides have risen. Then remove it from the oven.
6. While the pancake bakes, toss the blackberries and honey in a small bowl.
7. In a microwave-safe bowl, melt the white chocolate in the microwave for 20 seconds, stirring, and repeating 1 or 2 more times until smooth.

8. Cut the hot pancake into wedges. Top the slices with blackberries and a drizzle of white chocolate. Serve with maple syrup or honey for dipping.

18. Curry Scramble

Servings: 4
Cooking Time: 15 Min
Ingredients:
- 8 large eggs
- 1/4 cup fat-free milk
- 1/2 teaspoon curry powder
- 1/4 teaspoon salt
- 1/8 teaspoon pepper
- 1/8 teaspoon ground cardamom, optional
- 2 medium tomatoes, sliced or chopped

Directions:
1. In a large bowl, whisk the eggs, milk, curry powder, salt, pepper and, if desired, cardamom until blended.
2. Place a large nonstick skillet coated with cooking spray over medium heat. Pour in egg mixture; cook and stir until eggs are thickened and no liquid egg remains. Serve with tomatoes.

19. Peanut Butter And Banana Baked Oatmeal

Servings: 4
Cooking Time: 40 To 45 Minutes
Ingredients:
- 2 cups rolled oats
- 2 ripe bananas, sliced
- 1 tablespoon packed brown sugar
- 1 teaspoon baking powder
- ½ teaspoon sea salt
- 2 eggs
- 1½ cups whole milk
- ¼ cup honey
- 3 tablespoons salted butter, room temperature
- ½ cup smooth peanut butter

Directions:
1. Preheat the oven to 350°F.
2. In a large bowl, stir together the oats, bananas, brown sugar, baking powder, and salt.
3. In a medium bowl, whisk together the eggs, milk, honey, and butter.
4. Fold the milk mixture into the oat mixture. Spoon half of the batter into your skillet.
5. Swirl half of the peanut butter into the batter, then top with the remaining half.
6. Bake for 40 to 45 minutes or until crisp around the edges and cooked through. Serve hot.

20. Smoked Salmon And Goat Cheese Frittata

Servings: 6
Cooking Time: 15 To 20 Minutes
Ingredients:
- 2 tablespoons salted butter
- 1 white onion, chopped
- 2 garlic cloves, minced
- 6 eggs
- 1 cup crumbled goat cheese
- ¼ cup heavy cream
- Pinch sea salt
- 8 ounces smoked salmon, coarsely chopped

- 3 tablespoons minced fresh dill

Directions:
1.   Preheat the oven to 400°F.
2.   In your skillet, melt the butter over medium heat. Add the onions and garlic and cook for 3 to 5 minutes, stirring occasionally until the onions have begun to soften.
3.   In a large bowl, whisk together the eggs, cheese, cream, and salt.
4.   Stir the smoked salmon into the egg mixture and pour it into the skillet over the onions. Cook for 1 to 2 minutes or until the eggs begin to set. Transfer the skillet to the oven.
5.   Bake for 8 to 10 minutes, until the eggs have set.
6.   Top with the fresh dill and serve warm.

21.   Bacon And Cheese Frittata

Servings: 8 Servings
Cooking Time: 15 Minutes
Ingredients:
- 8 slices bacon, chopped
- 12 large eggs
- 3 tablespoons milk
- Coarse salt
- Freshly ground pepper
- ¼ cup Romano cheese
- ½ cup grated cheddar cheese
- Dash of hot sauce

Directions:
1.   Preheat oven to 375 degrees.
2.   Heat cast iron skillet and cook bacon over medium heat, stirring until crisp. Set aside on a plate.
3.   In a large bowl, whisk eggs, milk, salt, pepper, cheeses and hot sauce. Add cooked bacon to egg mixture. Pour eggs into cast iron skillet. When eggs are half set and edges begin to pull away, place frittata in oven and bake for about 10 minutes, or until center is no longer jiggly. Cut into wedges inside skillet or slide out of skillet onto serving plate.

Nutrition Info: Calories: 255, Sodium: 632 mg, Dietary Fiber: 0 g, Total Fat: 18.8 g, Total Carbs: 1.3 g, Protein: 19.5 g.

22.   Farmers Breakfast

Servings: 4-6
Cooking Time: 20 Min
Ingredients:
- 6 bacon strips, diced
- 2 tablespoons diced onion
- 3 medium potatoes, cooked and cubed
- 6 large eggs, beaten
- Salt and pepper to taste
- 1/2 cup shredded cheddar cheese

Directions:
1.   In a skillet, cook bacon until crisp. Remove to paper towel to drain. In drippings, saute onion and potatoes until potatoes are browned, about 5 minutes. Pour eggs into skillet; cook and stir gently until eggs are set and cooked to desired doneness. Season with salt and pepper. Sprinkle with cheese and bacon; let stand for 2-3 minutes or until cheese melts.

23.   Andouille And Bell Pepper Breakfast Hash

Servings: 4
Cooking Time: 35 Minutes
Ingredients:

- 8 ounces andouille sausage
- 1 tablespoon olive oil, for cooking
- 2 tablespoons salted butter
- 1 white onion, chopped
- 2 garlic cloves, minced
- 2 cups cubed red potatoes
- 1½ teaspoons Cajun seasoning
- ½ teaspoon sea salt
- 1 red bell pepper, cut into strips
- 1 green bell pepper, cut into strips
- 4 ounces Cheddar cheese, shredded

Directions:

1. Warm the skillet over medium heat. When it's hot, add the sausage and oil. Cook for 8 to 10 minutes, or until browned and crisp. Transfer the sausage to a plate, cut it into ½-inch slices, and set aside.
2. Put the butter, onion, and garlic into the skillet. Cook for 3 to 4 minutes, until the onion begins to soften. Add the potatoes, Cajun seasoning, and salt and stir thoroughly. Distribute the potatoes evenly in the skillet. Cook for 7 to 10 minutes, stirring occasionally, until they are browned and crisp.
3. Stir in the red and green bell peppers and cook for 5 to 7 minutes, until the potatoes are cooked through.
4. Stir the sausage slices into the potatoes. Remove the hash from the heat, sprinkle with the Cheddar cheese, and serve.

24. Creamy Eggs & Mushrooms Au Gratin

Servings: 8
Cooking Time: 25 Min
Ingredients:

- 2 tablespoons butter
- 1 pound sliced fresh mushrooms
- 1 green onion, chopped
- SAUCE
- 2 tablespoons butter, melted
- 3 tablespoons all-purpose flour
- 1/2 teaspoon salt
- 1/8 teaspoon pepper
- 1 cup 2% milk
- 1/2 cup heavy whipping cream
- 2 tablespoons grated Parmesan cheese
- EGGS
- 16 large eggs
- 1/4 teaspoon salt
- 1/8 teaspoon pepper
- 1/4 cup butter, cubed
- 1/2 cup grated Parmesan cheese
- 1 green onion, finely chopped

Directions:

1. In a large broiler-safe skillet, heat butter over medium-high heat. Add mushrooms; cook and stir 4-6 minutes or until browned. Add green onion; cook 1 minute longer. Remove from pan with a slotted spoon. Wipe skillet clean.
2. For sauce, in a small saucepan, melt butter over medium heat. Stir in flour, salt and pepper until smooth; whisk in milk and cream. Bring to a boil, stirring constantly; cook and stir 2-4 minutes or until thickened. Remove from heat; stir in cheese.
3. Preheat broiler. For eggs, in a large bowl, whisk eggs, salt and pepper until blended. In same skillet, heat butter over medium heat. Pour in egg mixture; cook and stir just until eggs are thickened and no liquid egg remains. Remove from heat.
4. Spoon half of the sauce over the eggs; top with mushrooms. Add remaining sauce; sprinkle with cheese. Broil 4-5 in. from heat 4-6 minutes or until top is lightly browned. Sprinkle with green onion.

25. Bananas Foster Dutch Baby

Servings: 2
Cooking Time: 25 Minutes
Ingredients:
- For the Dutch baby
- 1 cup buttermilk
- 3 large eggs
- 2 tablespoons granulated sugar
- 1 teaspoon vanilla extract
- Pinch sea salt
- ¾ cups all-purpose flour
- 5 tablespoons salted butter
- For the bananas Foster
- 6 tablespoons (¾ stick) salted butter
- ¾ cup packed light brown sugar
- 1 teaspoon vanilla extract
- ½ teaspoon ground cinnamon
- 2 tablespoons banana liqueur or creme de banana
- 2 ripe bananas, sliced
- ¼ cup dark rum
- For the whipped cream
- 1 cup heavy (whipping) cream
- 2 tablespoons granulated sugar
- 1 teaspoon vanilla extract

Directions:
1. To make the Dutch baby: Preheat the oven to 425°F. Adjust an oven rack to the middle position and place the 10-inch skillet on it while the oven preheats.
2. In a medium bowl, whisk the buttermilk, eggs, granulated sugar, vanilla, and salt to blend. Gently fold in the flour until blended. Let the batter rest for 5 minutes.
3. Using an oven mitt, remove the skillet from the oven. Melt the butter into the skillet, then swirl the skillet to coat.
4. Pour the batter into the skillet and immediately place it into the oven. Bake for 15 to 20 minutes, or until the Dutch baby is golden brown and the sides have risen.
5. To make the bananas Foster: While the Dutch baby bakes, melt the butter in the 12-inch skillet or a large saucepan over medium heat. Stir in the brown sugar, vanilla, and cinnamon and cook until the brown sugar dissolves.
6. Stir in the liqueur and bananas. Mix well and let it bubble for 1 to 2 minutes, or until thickened.
7. Add the rum, taking care not to drip it onto the hot stovetop. Using oven mitts, transfer the skillet to a heatproof surface. Use a stick lighter or torch to carefully light the bananas Foster, then watch from a safe distance as the alcohol burns off.
8. As the flames die down, return the skillet to the heat and resume stirring. Let the sauce thicken for 2 to 3 minutes. Remove from the heat.
9. To make the whipped cream: In the bowl of a stand mixer fitted with the whisk attachment or a large bowl using an electric mixer, combine the cream, granulated sugar, and vanilla. Beat on high speed until stiff peaks form.
10. Remove the Dutch baby from the oven. Top it with the bananas Foster and whipped cream, and serve.

26. Italian Egg Skillet

Servings: 2
Cooking Time: 10 Minutes
Ingredients:
- ½ tbsp. butter
- ½ cup mushrooms, sliced
- 3 cups raw baby spinach
- ¾ cup marinara sauce
- 4 eggs

- 2 tbsps. mozzarella cheese, shredded
- Salt and pepper to taste

Directions:
1. Melt the butter in the skillet. Add mushrooms and cook for 5 minutes.
2. Add the spinach and cook for 1 minute.
3. Stir in marinara sauce and mix to combine.
4. Crack eggs evenly over the top of the vegetables and cover with a lid. Cook until egg whites are set.
5. Remove the lid and sprinkle with cheese, salt, and pepper. Serve.

27. Sweet Potato And Egg Hash

Servings: 2
Cooking Time: 6 Minutes
Ingredients:
- 1 large sweet potato, cut into cubes
- ½ cup fresh spinach leaves
- 2 eggs
- ½ tsp cinnamon
- ½ tsp garlic powder
- 2 tbsps. of oil
- Salt and pepper to taste

Directions:
1. Grease the skillet with oil and add the sweet potato cubes. Season with the cinnamon and garlic powder and sauté for 3 minutes.
2. Add the spinach and cook for 1 minute more.
3. Crack the eggs on top and season with salt and pepper. Cover with a lid for 2 minutes to cook the eggs.
4. Serve.

28. Apple Dutch Baby Pancake

Servings: 4-6 Servings
Cooking Time: 20 Minutes
Ingredients:
- 3 large eggs, room temperature
- ¾ cup whole milk
- ¾ cup all-purpose flour
- 1 teaspoon almond extract
- ¼ teaspoon salt
- 2 large Granny Smith apples, peeled, cored and sliced
- 1 tablespoon sugar
- 1 teaspoon cinnamon
- ½ teaspoon ginger
- 4 tablespoons butter, divided
- 2 tablespoons light brown sugar

Directions:
1. Preheat oven to 400 degrees.
2. Whisk together eggs, milk, flour, extract and salt.
3. Place sliced apples in a bowl with sugar, cinnamon and ginger.
4. Melt 2 tablespoons butter in heated cast iron skillet. Sprinkle brown sugar inside skillet. Add apples and cook until apples have softened. Transfer to plate.
5. Wipe out skillet and melt remaining 2 tablespoons butter. Make sure to coat sides of skillet as well. When skillet is very hot, add apples and pour batter inside skillet. Bake until puffed and golden, about 13-15 minutes.

Nutrition Info: Calories: 240, Sodium: 201 mg, Dietary Fiber: 2.4 g, Total Fat: 11.4 g, Total Carbs: 29.2 g, Protein: 6.0 g.

29. Spicy Shakshuka

Servings: 2
Cooking Time: 10 Servings
Ingredients:
- 4 whole eggs
- 1 ½ cups tomato sauce
- 1 scallion, chopped
- ½ tsp garlic powder
- ½ tsp nutmeg
- ½ tsp cumin
- 1 tsp smoked paprika
- ½ tsp cayenne pepper
- 3 tbsp olive oil
- ½ tsp sugar
- Salt to taste
- Chopped parsley for garnish

Directions:
1. Heat the oil in a skillet and add the chopped scallion. Cook for 3 minutes.
2. Add the tomato sauce and all the seasonings with salt and sugar. Mix and crack the eggs on top of the mixture.
3. Cover the skillet with a lid and cook the eggs for 2 minutes.
4. Garnish and serve.

30. Cinnamon-sugar French Toast

Servings: 4 Servings
Cooking Time: 5 Minutes
Ingredients:
- 1 cup whole milk
- 4 eggs
- 1 teaspoon cinnamon
- 1/8 teaspoon nutmeg
- 1/8 teaspoon ground cloves
- 2 tablespoons sugar
- Pinch of salt
- 8-10 slices French bread
- 2 tablespoons unsalted butter

Directions:
1. Beat together the milk, eggs, cinnamon, nutmeg, cloves, sugar and salt.
2. Heat a cast iron skillet to medium heat.
3. Dredge bread inside egg mixture, turning over several times.
4. Add butter to cast iron skillet and melt until foaming. Lay bread slices inside skillet and cook 2-3 minutes on each side, until browned. Sprinkle with additional cinnamon-sugar or serve with maple syrup.

Nutrition Info: Calories: 406, Sodium: 647 mg, Dietary Fiber: 2.3 g, Total Fat: 13.6 g, Total Carbs: 54.8 g, Protein: 17.0 g.

31. Bacon N' Eggs Skillet Breakfast

Servings: 4 Servings
Cooking Time: 15 Minutes
Ingredients:
- 4 strips bacon, chopped
- 1 small onion, finely chopped
- 3 medium, potatoes, boiled and cut into cubes
- 1 tomato, diced
- 6 eggs, beaten

- 2 tablespoons milk
- Salt and pepper
- ½ cup mozzarella cheese
- Dash hot pepper sauce

Directions:
1. In a cast iron skillet, fry bacon until crisp, 3-4 minutes. Transfer to a plate. Leave bacon fat in skillet.
2. Add onion and sauté until onion softens, 3-4 minutes. Brown potatoes with onion, another 5 minutes. Add diced tomato. Transfer to plate with bacon.
3. Combine eggs and milk in a bowl and pour into skillet. Season with salt and pepper. Transfer bacon and vegetables into skillet and top with cheese. Let stand on burner until cheese melts. Add a pinch of hot pepper sauce.

Nutrition Info: Calories: 374, Sodium: 631 mg, Dietary Fiber: 4.1 g, Total Fat: 17.3 g, Total Carbs: 31.8 g, Protein: 23.2 g.

32. Upside-down Apple Cake

Servings: 6
Cooking Time: 45 Minutes
Ingredients:
- FOR THE APPLES
- ½ cup brown sugar
- 1 stick salted butter
- 4 or 5 Granny Smith apples, peeled, cored, and cut into slices
- FOR THE CAKE
- 1 stick salted butter, room temperature
- ¾ cup granulated sugar
- 2 eggs
- 1 teaspoon vanilla extract
- 1½ cups all-purpose flour
- ½ teaspoon baking soda
- 1 teaspoon baking powder
- ½ teaspoon sea salt
- ¾ cup Greek yogurt
- Honey for drizzling

Directions:
1. Preheat the oven to 375°F.
2. In your skillet, combine the brown sugar and butter over medium heat. Stir well and then place the apples into the skillet, making sure the slices are lying flat on their sides.
3. Lower the heat to a simmer and allow the mixture to caramelize.
4. In a large bowl, using a handheld mixer or a stand mixer, cream the butter and sugar.
5. Add in the eggs, one at a time, mixing in each egg completely before adding the next.
6. Add in the vanilla.
7. In a separate bowl, mix together the flour, baking soda, baking powder, and salt. Add the dry mixture to the wet batter ⅓ at a time, alternating with adding the Greek yogurt ¼ cup at a time.
8. Mix well, making sure to scrape the bottom of the bowl to catch any pockets of flour.
9. Remove the skillet from the heat when the apples start to brown and soften. Spoon the batter over the apples.
10. Bake for 20 to 25 minutes, until the cake is cooked through and golden brown.
11. Allow to cool in the skillet for 5 minutes before turning the cake out onto your serving dish.
12. Top with a drizzle of honey and serve.

33. Italian Sausage Breakfast Wraps

Servings: 6
Cooking Time: 30 Min
Ingredients:
- 3/4 pound Italian turkey sausage links, casings removed

- 1 small green pepper, finely chopped
- 1 small onion, finely chopped
- 1 medium tomato, chopped
- 4 large eggs
- 6 large egg whites
- 1 cup chopped fresh spinach
- 6 whole wheat tortillas (8 inches)
- 1 cup (4 ounces) shredded reduced-fat cheddar cheese

Directions:

1. In a large skillet, cook sausage, pepper, onion and tomato over medium heat until meat is no longer pink and vegetables are tender, breaking up sausage into crumbles; drain. Return to pan.

2. In a bowl, whisk eggs and egg whites until blended. Add egg mixture to sausage. Cook and stir until eggs are thickened and no liquid egg remains. Add spinach; cook and stir just until wilted.

3. Spoon 3/4 cup egg mixture across center of each tortilla; top with about 2 tablespoons cheese. Fold bottom and sides of tortilla over filling and roll up.

FISH & SEAFOOD RECIPES

34. Brown Butter And Garlic Wahoo

Servings: 4
Cooking Time: 40 Minutes
Ingredients:
- 8 tablespoons (1 stick) salted butter
- 2 garlic cloves, minced
- 1 lemon, sliced
- 4 wahoo steaks
- Pinch sea salt

Directions:
1. In the skillet over medium-low heat, melt the butter.
2. Add the garlic and 3 or 4 lemon slices, and let the butter come to a simmer. Cook for 30 minutes, stirring occasionally, until the butter is golden brown.
3. Season the wahoo steaks with salt. Increase the heat under the skillet to medium-high. Sear the wahoo for 3 to 4 minutes per side.
4. Top with a squeeze of fresh lemon and serve with lemon slices on the side.

35. Skillet-grilled Catfish

Servings: 4
Cooking Time: 25 Min
Ingredients:
- 1/4 cup all-purpose flour
- 1/4 cup cornmeal
- 1 teaspoon onion powder
- 1 teaspoon dried basil
- 1/2 teaspoon garlic salt
- 1/2 teaspoon dried thyme
- 1/4 to 1/2 teaspoon white pepper
- 1/4 to 1/2 teaspoon cayenne pepper
- 1/4 to 1/2 teaspoon pepper
- 4 catfish fillets (6 to 8 ounces each)
- 1/4 cup butter

Directions:
1. In a large resealable bag, combine the first nine ingredients. Add catfish, one fillet at a time, and shake to coat.
2. Place a large cast-iron skillet on a grill rack over medium-hot heat. Melt butter in the skillet; add catfish. Grill, covered, for 5-10 minutes on each side or until fish flakes easily with a fork.

36. Seared Ahi Tuna

Servings: 2
Cooking Time: 5 Minutes
Ingredients:
- Juice of 1 lime
- 2 tablespoons soy sauce
- 1 tablespoon sesame oil, plus 1 teaspoon
- 1 teaspoon honey
- 2 tablespoons minced garlic
- 1 tablespoon peeled, grated fresh ginger
- 1 tablespoon minced scallion
- 2 tuna steaks
- 1 tablespoon white sesame seeds
- 1 tablespoon black sesame seeds

- Pinch sea salt
- 1 teaspoon vegetable oil

Directions:
1. In a small bowl, whisk the lime juice, soy sauce, 1 tablespoon of sesame oil, honey, garlic, ginger, and scallion to combine. Set the sauce aside.
2. Pat the tuna dry and sprinkle both sides with white and black sesame seeds and salt.
3. Heat the vegetable oil and the remaining 1 teaspoon of sesame oil in the skillet over high heat. Sear the tuna for 1 to 2 minutes per side for rare and 2 to 3 minutes per side for medium. Remove the tuna from the heat and let it rest on a cutting board for 5 minutes.
4. Slice the tuna, put it on plates, and drizzle sauce over the top.

37. Salmon With Peach Chutney

Servings: 2
Cooking Time: 1 Hour
Ingredients:
- 2 skinned salmon fillets, fresh or thawed from frozen
- 1 ½ (15 oz.) cans sliced peaches in pure juice, drained and cubed
- 1/3 cup brown sugar
- 1 red onion, chopped
- ¼ tsp garlic powder
- ¼ tsp ground cumin
- 1 tbsp lime juice
- ¼ cup white vinegar
- 1 tbsp vegetable oil
- Salt and pepper to taste

Directions:
1. To make the chutney, combine the peaches, brown sugar, vinegar, onion, and spices. Bring to a boil. Lower heat and simmer for 40 minutes, stirring 2 times.
2. Add the lime juice and simmer for 10 minutes more.
3. Season the salmon fillets with salt and pepper and heat the oil in the skillet. Cook for 3 minutes on each side (for medium to well-done).
4. Add the peach chutney and cook covered for 3 minutes.
5. Rest for 5 minutes and serve.

38. Rustic Crusted Salmon

Servings: 2
Cooking Time: 20 Minutes
Ingredients:
- 2 tbsps. unsalted butter
- 18 butter crackers, crushed
- 1 tbsp. minced fresh parsley
- Salt and pepper to taste
- 2 (6-ounce) salmon fillets, skin on
- 1 tbsp. olive oil
- ½ lemon, cut into wedges, for serving

Directions:
1. Melt the butter in a bowl.
2. In another bowl, mix the crackers, parsley, and salt and pepper to taste.
3. Brush the tops of the salmon fillets with melted butter and press the cracker mixture into the butter.
4. Heat the oil in the skillet until very hot.
5. Add the salmon and sear it, skin-side down for 5 minutes, or until the skin is brown.
6. Move to low heat, cover, and cook for 5 to 10 minutes more or until the salmon is almost cooked through.
7. Remove from the heat and let it rest, covered for 5 minutes. Serve with lemon wedges.

39. Blackened Catfish With Mango Avocado Salsa

Servings: 4 (2 Cups Salsa)
Cooking Time: 10 Min
Ingredients:
- 2 teaspoons dried oregano
- 2 teaspoons ground cumin
- 2 teaspoons paprika
- 2 1/4 teaspoons pepper, divided
- 3/4 teaspoon salt, divided
- 4 catfish fillets (6 ounces each)
- 1 medium mango, peeled and cubed
- 1 medium ripe avocado, peeled and cubed
- 1/3 cup finely chopped red onion
- 2 tablespoons minced fresh cilantro
- 2 tablespoons lime juice
- 2 teaspoons olive oil

Directions:
1. Combine the oregano, cumin, paprika, 2 teaspoons pepper and 1/2 teaspoon salt; rub over fillets. Refrigerate for at least 30 minutes.
2. Meanwhile, in a small bowl, combine the mango, avocado, red onion, cilantro, lime juice and remaining salt and pepper. Chill until serving.
3. In a large cast-iron skillet, cook fillets in oil over medium heat for 5-7 minutes on each side or until fish flakes easily with a fork. Serve with salsa.

40. Blackened Mahi-mahi Tacos With Mango Salsa

Servings: 4
Cooking Time: 10 Minutes
Ingredients:
- For the salsa
- 3 mangos, peeled and diced
- 1 cup cherry tomatoes, quartered
- 1 green bell pepper, diced
- 1 jalapeño pepper, seeded and minced
- ½ red onion, diced
- Juice of 2 limes
- 1 tablespoon white wine vinegar
- Handful fresh cilantro, minced
- Sea salt
- Freshly ground black pepper
- For the tacos
- 1 teaspoon dried oregano
- 1 teaspoon freshly ground black pepper
- 1 teaspoon sea salt
- 1 teaspoon smoked paprika
- ½ teaspoon cayenne
- ¼ teaspoon red pepper flakes
- ¼ teaspoon ground cumin
- 4 mahi steaks
- 4 tablespoons (½ stick) salted butter, melted
- 8 flour tortillas or 12 corn tortillas
- 1 cup shredded cabbage
- 2 limes, cut into wedges
- Sour cream, for serving (optional)

Directions:

1.   To make the salsa: Begin by making the salsa so it has time for the flavors to blend. In a large bowl, stir together the mangos, tomatoes, bell pepper, jalapeño, onion, lime juice, vinegar, cilantro, and salt and pepper to taste. Set aside in the refrigerator.
2.   To make the tacos: In a small bowl, stir together the oregano, black pepper, salt, paprika, cayenne, red pepper flakes, and cumin. Set aside.
3.   Heat the skillet over medium-high heat.
4.   Brush both sides of each fish fillet with melted butter and carefully coat both sides with the spice mixture.
5.   Place the fillets in the hot skillet and cook for 2 to 3 minutes per side, until blackened and cooked through. Let the mahi rest for 2 to 3 minutes, then slice or roughly chop.
6.   Layer each tortilla with mahi, cabbage, and salsa. Serve with a lime wedge and sour cream (if using).

41. Shrimp Burgers With Chipotle Mayonnaise

Servings: 4
Cooking Time: 10 Minutes
Ingredients:
- 1 pound shrimp, peeled and deveined
- ¼ cup bread crumbs
- 1 large egg, beaten
- 2 shallots, minced
- 2 garlic cloves, minced
- ¼ cup fresh cilantro, roughly chopped
- Juice of 1½ lemons, divided
- Sea salt
- ¼ cup mayonnaise
- 1 teaspoon chipotle powder
- 2 tablespoons olive oil
- 4 hamburger buns, toasted
- Lettuce, for topping

Directions:
1.   Divide the shrimp into thirds. Finely mince one third, dice one third, and roughly chop one third. Put all the shrimp into a large bowl.
2.   Stir in the bread crumbs, egg, shallots, garlic, cilantro, juice of 1 lemon, and a pinch of salt. Divide and form the shrimp mixture into 4 patties. Gently place the patties on a plate and chill for 25 minutes.
3.   In a small bowl, stir together the mayonnaise, remaining juice of ½ lemon, the chipotle powder, and a pinch of salt. Set aside.
4.   Heat the oil in the skillet over medium-high heat. Place the patties into the skillet and cook for 4 to 5 minutes, or until browned. Flip and cook for 3 to 4 minutes more.
5.   Spread the chipotle mayonnaise evenly on the cut side of each bun. Top each bottom bun with a shrimp burger and lettuce, then serve.

42. Blackened Halibut

Servings: 4
Cooking Time: 25 Min
Ingredients:
- 2 tablespoons garlic powder
- 1 tablespoon salt
- 1 tablespoon onion powder
- 1 tablespoon dried oregano
- 1 tablespoon dried thyme
- 1 tablespoon cayenne pepper
- 1 tablespoon pepper
- 2 1/2 teaspoons paprika
- 4 halibut fillets (4 ounces each)
- 2 tablespoons butter

Directions:

1. In a large resealable plastic bag, combine the first eight ingredients. Add fillets, two at a time, and shake to coat.
2. In a large cast-iron skillet, cook the fillets in butter over medium heat for 3-4 minutes on each side or until fish flakes easily with a fork.

43. Feta Shrimp Skillet

Servings: 4
Cooking Time: 30 Min
Ingredients:
- 1 tablespoon olive oil
- 1 medium onion, finely chopped
- 3 garlic cloves, minced
- 1 teaspoon dried oregano
- 1/2 teaspoon pepper
- 1/4 teaspoon salt
- 2 cans (14 1/2 ounces each) diced tomatoes, undrained
- 1/4 cup white wine, optional
- 1 pound uncooked medium shrimp, peeled and deveined
- 2 tablespoons minced fresh parsley
- 3/4 cup crumbled feta cheese

Directions:
1. In a large nonstick skillet, heat oil over medium-high heat. Add onion; cook and stir 4-6 minutes or until tender. Add garlic and seasonings; cook 1 minute longer. Stir in tomatoes and, if desired, wine. Bring to a boil. Reduce the heat; simmer, uncovered, for 5-7 minutes or until the sauce is slightly thickened.
2. Add the shrimp and parsley; cook 5-6 minutes or until shrimp turn pink, stirring occasionally. Remove from heat; sprinkle with cheese. Let stand, covered, until cheese is softened.

44. Seared Lobster Tails

Servings: 2
Cooking Time: 10 Minutes
Ingredients:
- 2 lobster tails, cleaned
- Pinch sea salt
- Pinch freshly ground black pepper
- Pinch red pepper flakes
- Juice of 1 lemon, divided
- 2 tablespoons olive oil
- 2 tablespoons salted butter
- 2 garlic cloves, minced
- 2 tablespoons fresh parsley leaves, minced

Directions:
1. Season the meat side of the lobster with salt, black pepper, and red pepper flakes. Squeeze half of the lemon juice over the lobster.
2. Heat the oil and melt the butter in the skillet over medium-high heat. Add the garlic.
3. Put the lobster in the skillet, meat-side down, and cook for 2 to 3 minutes, or until the meat is crisp and golden brown. Flip the lobster, cover the skillet, and cook for 2 to 3 minutes more, until the lobster meat is opaque and the shells have turned red. Remove the tails from the heat.
4. Top with the remaining half of the lemon juice and the parsley and serve.

45. Spicy Sriracha Shrimps

Servings: 2
Cooking Time: 8 Minutes
Ingredients:

- ½ lb. raw frozen shrimps, peeled and thawed
- 1/6 cup sriracha sauce
- ½ tbsp. butter, melted
- ½ tbsp. barbeque sauce

Directions:
1. Heat the butter in the skillet and add the shrimps. Cook for 2 minutes.
2. Add the sriracha and barbeque sauce and cook for 3 minutes. Serve.

46. Lemon-pepper Tilapia With Mushrooms

Servings: 4
Cooking Time: 25 Min
Ingredients:
- 2 tablespoons butter
- 1/2 pound sliced fresh mushrooms
- 3/4 teaspoon lemon-pepper seasoning, divided
- 3 garlic cloves, minced
- 4 tilapia fillets (6 ounces each)
- 1/4 teaspoon paprika
- 1/8 teaspoon cayenne pepper
- 1 medium tomato, chopped
- 3 green onions, thinly sliced

Directions:
1. In a 12-in. skillet, heat the butter over medium heat. Add mushrooms and 1/4 teaspoon lemon pepper; cook and stir 3-5 minutes or until mushrooms are tender. Add the garlic; cook 30 seconds longer.
2. Place fillets over mushrooms; sprinkle with paprika, cayenne and remaining lemon pepper. Cook, covered, 5-7 minutes or until fish just begins to flake easily with a fork. Top with tomato and green onions.

47. Mediterranean-style Red Snapper

Servings: 4
Cooking Time: 30 Min
Ingredients:
- 1 teaspoon lemon-pepper seasoning
- 1/2 teaspoon garlic powder
- 1/2 teaspoon dried thyme
- 1/8 teaspoon cayenne pepper
- 4 red snapper fillets (6 ounces each)
- 2 teaspoons olive oil, divided
- 1/2 medium sweet red pepper, julienned
- 3 green onions, chopped
- 1 garlic clove, minced
- 1 can (14 1/2 ounces) diced tomatoes, undrained
- 1/2 cup chopped pimiento-stuffed olives
- 1/4 cup chopped ripe olives
- 1/4 cup minced chives

Directions:
1. Combine the lemon pepper, garlic powder, thyme and cayenne; rub over fillets. In a large nonstick skillet coated with cooking spray, cook fillets in 1 teaspoon oil over medium heat for 4-5 minutes on each side or until fish flakes easily with a fork. Remove and keep warm.
2. In the same pan, saute the red pepper and onions in remaining oil until crisp-tender. Add garlic; cook 1 minute longer. Stir in tomatoes. Bring to a boil. Reduce heat; simmer, uncovered, for 3 minutes or until liquid has evaporated. Serve with snapper. Sprinkle with olives and chives.

48. Bacon-wrapped Scallops

Servings: 4
Cooking Time: 20 Minutes
Ingredients:
- 12 large sea scallops
- 6 thin-cut bacon strips, halved lengthwise
- Pinch sea salt
- 1 tablespoon olive oil
- 2 tablespoons salted butter, divided
- 2 garlic cloves, minced
- Juice of 1 lemon

Directions:
1. Preheat the oven to 425°F. Place the skillet into the oven to preheat.
2. Pat the scallops dry. Wrap a halved bacon strip around each scallop, securing it with a toothpick. Season the scallops with salt.
3. Using oven mitts, remove the skillet from the oven and put the oil and 1 tablespoon of butter into the skillet. Stir or swirl the skillet to combine.
4. Place the wrapped scallops into the skillet and return it to the oven. Bake for 15 to 17 minutes.
5. Using oven mitts, remove the skillet from the oven and add the remaining 1 tablespoon of butter and the garlic and flip the scallops. Let them cook in the hot skillet for 2 to 3 minutes. Top with lemon juice and serve hot.

49. Pineapple Shrimp Stir-fry

Servings: 4
Cooking Time: 30 Min
Ingredients:
- 1 can (20 ounces) unsweetened pineapple tidbits
- 2 tablespoons cornstarch
- 1 cup chicken broth
- 1 tablespoon brown sugar
- 1 tablespoon orange juice
- 1 tablespoon reduced-sodium soy sauce
- 1 tablespoon sesame or canola oil
- 1 medium sweet red pepper, thinly sliced
- 1 medium green pepper, thinly sliced
- 1 medium sweet onion, thinly sliced
- 1 pound uncooked shrimp (31-40 per pound), peeled and deveined
- 1/4 cup flaked coconut, toasted
- Hot cooked rice

Directions:
1. Drain pineapple, reserving juice. In a small bowl, mix cornstarch, broth, brown sugar, orange juice, soy sauce and reserved pineapple juice until the mixture is smooth.
2. In a large skillet, heat oil over medium-high heat. Add peppers and onion; stir-fry 1-2 minutes or just until crisp-tender. Add shrimp; stir-fry 2-3 minutes longer or until shrimp turn pink. Remove from pan.
3. Place pineapple in skillet. Stir the cornstarch mixture and add to pan. Bring to a boil; cook and stir 4-5 minutes or until sauce is thickened. Return shrimp mixture to pan; heat through, stirring to combine. Sprinkle with coconut; serve with rice.

50. Seafood Jambalaya

Servings: 4
Cooking Time: 45 Minutes
Ingredients:
- 1 tablespoon olive oil
- 1 pound andouille sausage, cut into ½-inch slices
- 3 celery stalks, roughly chopped

- 1 green bell pepper, chopped
- 1 white onion, chopped
- 2 teaspoons Cajun seasoning
- ½ teaspoon sea salt
- 8 ounces catfish, diced
- 4 Roma tomatoes, chopped
- 3 garlic cloves, minced
- 1 cup long-grain white rice, rinsed
- 2 cups chicken broth or seafood broth
- 1 pound shrimp, peeled and deveined
- Handful fresh cilantro, minced
- 2 lemons, cut into wedges

Directions:
1. Heat the oil in the skillet over medium heat. Cook the sausage for 3 to 4 minutes per side, until it begins to brown. Add the celery, bell pepper, and onion. Cook for 7 to 9 minutes, stirring frequently, until the vegetables begin to caramelize.
2. Stir in the Cajun seasoning, salt, catfish, tomatoes, and garlic. Cook for 2 to 3 minutes.
3. Stir in the rice, then add the broth. Bring to a boil, then reduce the heat to low, cover the skillet, and simmer for 20 to 25 minutes, or until the rice absorbs most of the liquid. Stir in the shrimp. Cook for 3 to 4 minutes. Remove from heat and uncover. Stir and let rest for 10 minutes.
4. Top with cilantro and serve with lemon wedges.

51. Seared Breaded Cod With Corn & Tomato Salsa

Servings: 2
Cooking Time: 15 Minutes
Ingredients:
- 2 fillets of cod (fresh or thawed from Frozen)
- 2 eggs, beaten
- ¼ cup flour
- ¼ cup Italian seasoning breadcrumbs
- ¾ cup cherry tomatoes, halved
- ¼ cup sweet corn kernels
- ¼ cup olive oil
- ½ tbsp oregano
- 1 tbsp dried parsley flakes
- ½ tbsp vinegar
- Salt and pepper to taste

Directions:
1. Keep the eggs, flour, and Italian style breadcrumbs in a separate bowl. Season the fillets lightly with the salt and pepper and dip each fillet into the flour first, then the egg wash, and lastly coat with the breadcrumbs.
2. Meanwhile, heat the oil in the skillet and add the cod fillets, and shallow fry until golden brown.
3. Remove from the heat and set aside. Keep only a few tbsp. of the oil.
4. In the same skillet with the remaining oil, add the tomatoes, with sweet corn, vinegar, parsley, and salt and pepper. Cook for 5 minutes.
5. Add the cod on top of the tomato and corn mixture and serve.

52. Cilantro Shrimp & Rice

Servings: 8
Cooking Time: 30 Min
Ingredients:
- 2 packages (8 1/2 ounces each) ready-to-serve basmati rice
- 2 tablespoons olive oil
- 2 cups frozen corn, thawed
- 2 medium zucchini, quartered and sliced
- 1 large sweet red pepper, chopped

- 1/2 teaspoon crushed red pepper flakes
- 3 garlic cloves, minced
- 1 pound peeled and deveined cooked large shrimp, tails removed
- 1/2 cup chopped fresh cilantro
- 1 tablespoon grated lime peel
- 2 tablespoons lime juice
- 3/4 teaspoon salt
- Lime wedges, optional

Directions:
1. Prepare rice according to package directions.
2. Meanwhile, in a large skillet, heat oil over medium-high heat. Add corn, zucchini, red pepper and pepper flakes; cook and stir 3-5 minutes or until zucchini is crisp-tender. Add garlic; cook 1 minute longer. Add shrimp; cook and stir 3-5 minutes or until heated through.
3. Stir in rice, cilantro, lime peel, lime juice and salt. If desired, serve with lime wedges.

53. Maple-glazed Salmon

Servings: 2
Cooking Time: 20 Minutes
Ingredients:
- 2 tablespoons soy sauce
- 1 tablespoon maple syrup
- 2 garlic cloves, minced
- 1 tablespoon peeled, minced fresh ginger
- Juice of 1 lime
- ¼ teaspoon paprika
- 1 tablespoon olive oil
- 2 (4-ounce) salmon fillets

Directions:
1. In a small bowl, whisk the soy sauce, maple syrup, garlic, ginger, lime juice, and paprika to combine.
2. Preheat the oven to 375°F.
3. Spread the oil evenly over the bottom of the skillet. Place the salmon into the skillet, skin-side down. Reserve 2 tablespoons of the sauce, then spoon what remains over the salmon.
4. Bake for 15 minutes, or until the salmon begins to brown and the flesh is opaque.
5. Using oven mitts, remove the salmon from the oven. Set the broiler to high.
6. Spoon the reserved sauce over the salmon. Return the salmon to the oven and broil for 2 to 3 minutes, or until a golden crust forms on the salmon. Remove from the oven and serve.

54. Halibut Steaks With Papaya Mint Salsa

Servings: 4
Cooking Time: 20 Min
Ingredients:
- 1 medium papaya, peeled, seeded and chopped
- 1/4 cup chopped red onion
- 1/4 cup fresh mint leaves
- 1 teaspoon finely chopped chipotle pepper in adobo sauce
- 2 tablespoons olive oil, divided
- 1 tablespoon honey
- 4 halibut steaks (6 ounces each)

Directions:
1. In a small bowl, combine the papaya, onion, mint, chipotle pepper, 1 tablespoon oil and honey. Cover and refrigerate until serving.
2. In a large skillet, cook halibut in remaining oil for 4-6 minutes on each side or until fish flakes easily with a fork. Serve with salsa.

55. Cornmeal Catfish With Avocado Sauce

Servings: 4 (3/4 Cup Sauce)
Cooking Time: 25 Min
Ingredients:
- 1 medium ripe avocado, peeled and cubed
- 1/3 cup reduced-fat mayonnaise
- 1/4 cup fresh cilantro leaves
- 2 tablespoons lime juice
- 1/2 teaspoon garlic salt
- 1/4 cup cornmeal
- 1 teaspoon seafood seasoning
- 4 catfish fillets (6 ounces each)
- 3 tablespoons canola oil
- 1 medium tomato, chopped

Directions:
1. Place the first five ingredients in a food processor; process until blended.
2. In a shallow bowl, mix the cornmeal and seafood seasoning. Dip the catfish in the cornmeal mixture to coat both sides; shake off excess.
3. In a large skillet, heat oil over medium heat. Add catfish in batches; cook 4-5 minutes on each side or until fish flakes easily with a fork. Top with avocado sauce and tomato.

56. Shrimp And Scallop Scampi

Servings: 4
Cooking Time: 15 Minutes
Ingredients:
- 1 pound angel hair pasta
- 6 tablespoons salted butter, divided
- 1 pound shrimp, peeled and deveined
- 3 garlic cloves, minced, divided
- Pinch sea salt
- 8 to 12 fresh sea scallops
- ½ cup dry white wine
- Juice of 1 lemon
- Handful fresh basil leaves

Directions:
1. Bring a large pot of salted water to a boil. Cook the angel hair pasta according to the package directions.
2. Meanwhile, in the skillet over medium heat, melt 2 tablespoons of butter. Put the shrimp, half of the garlic, and salt into the skillet. Cook the shrimp for 4 to 5 minutes, stirring occasionally, until the shrimp are pink. Remove from the skillet and set aside.
3. Add 2 tablespoons of butter to the skillet to melt. Put the scallops and the remaining garlic into the skillet. Sprinkle the scallops with salt and cook for 2 minutes. Flip and cook for 1 minute.
4. Return the shrimp to the skillet and pour in the wine and lemon juice. Cook for 2 minutes, stir in the basil, then remove from the heat.
5. Drain the pasta, return it to the pot, and toss it with the remaining 2 tablespoons of butter. Stir in the shrimp, scallops, and garlic butter from the skillet. Toss well and serve.

57. Shrimp And Grits

Servings: 4
Cooking Time: 50 Minutes
Ingredients:
- For the grits
- 4 cups water
- 2 cups yellow stone-ground grits
- 3 cups whole milk

- 2 teaspoons sea salt
- 1 teaspoon ground white pepper
- 1 teaspoon freshly ground black pepper
- 2 tablespoons salted butter
- ½ cup grated Parmesan cheese
- Juice of 1 lemon
- For the shrimp
- 8 ounces thick-cut bacon, roughly chopped
- 4 tablespoons (½ stick) salted butter
- 1 yellow onion, chopped
- 3 garlic cloves, minced
- 1 teaspoon red pepper flakes
- Pinch sea salt
- 1 pound shrimp, peeled and deveined
- Juice of 1 lemon
- ¼ cup roughly chopped scallion

Directions:
1.   To make the grits: In a medium pot over high heat, combine the water and grits. Bring to a boil, then reduce the heat to low.
2.   Stir in the milk, salt, white pepper, black pepper, and butter. Simmer for 40 to 45 minutes, stirring frequently, as the grits thicken.
3.   When the grits have absorbed the liquid (but still stir easily), stir in the Parmesan cheese and lemon juice. Remove from the heat.
4.   To make the shrimp: About 20 minutes before the grits are ready, put the bacon into the skillet, place it over medium heat, and cook for 8 to 10 minutes, stirring occasionally, or until it begins to brown and crisp.
5.   Add the butter, onion, garlic, red pepper flakes, and salt. Cook for 5 to 7 minutes, stirring frequently, until the onion begins to brown and soften.
6.   Add the shrimp to the skillet. Cook for 4 to 5 minutes, stirring frequently, until the shrimp turn pink. Sprinkle with lemon juice.
7.   Fill each bowl with a heaping serving of grits, then top with a generous portion of shrimp and bacon, making sure to get some of the pan juices, and finish with scallion.

58. Tuna Noodle Skillet

Servings: 6
Cooking Time: 30 Min
Ingredients:
- 2 jars (16 ounces each) Alfredo sauce
- 1 can (14 1/2 ounces) chicken broth
- 1 package (16 ounces) wide egg noodles
- 1 package (10 ounces) frozen peas
- 1/4 teaspoon pepper
- 1 can (12 ounces) albacore white tuna in water

Directions:
1.   In a large skillet over medium heat, bring Alfredo sauce and broth to a boil. Add noodles; cover and cook for 7-8 minutes.
2.   Reduce the heat; stir in the peas and pepper. Cover and cook 4 minutes longer or until the noodles are tender. Stir in tuna; heat through.

59. Mussels Steamed In Broth

Servings: 2
Cooking Time: 10 Minutes
Ingredients:
- ½ cup bottled clam juice
- ½ cup unsweetened coconut milk
- Finely grated zest of ½ lime

- ¾ tsp. rice vinegar
- ¾ tsp. sugar
- Salt to taste
- 1 tbsp. extra-virgin olive oil
- ¼ tsp. sesame oil
- ½ stalk fresh lemongrass, white part only, finely grated
- 1 garlic clove, minced
- 1 (1/2-inch) piece fresh ginger, peeled and minced
- ½ tbsp. chopped scallion (green parts only)
- ½ tbsp. chopped shallot
- ¼ tsp. red pepper flakes
- 1-pound live mussels in their shells, scrubbed and rinsed
- ¼ cup coarsely chopped fresh cilantro

Directions:
1. In a bowl, stir together the clam juice, coconut milk, lime zest, vinegar, sugar, and salt.
2. Heat the olive and sesame oils in a skillet. Add the lemongrass, garlic, ginger, scallion, shallot, and red pepper flakes, and cook for 15 seconds.
3. Add the clam juice mixture and bring to a boil. Add the mussels and stir to coat.
4. Cover the skillet and cook until most of the mussels open, about 5 minutes. Discard any mussels that do not open.
5. Garnish and serve.

60. Snapper With Zucchini & Mushrooms

Servings: 4
Cooking Time: 10 Min
Ingredients:
- 3 cups diced zucchini
- 2 cups halved fresh mushrooms
- 3/4 cup chopped sweet onion
- 2 tablespoons olive oil, divided
- 3 garlic cloves, minced
- 1 can (14 1/2 ounces) diced tomatoes, undrained
- 2 teaspoons minced fresh basil or 1/2 teaspoon dried basil
- 2 teaspoons minced fresh oregano or 1/2 teaspoon dried oregano
- 1/4 teaspoon salt
- 1/4 teaspoon pepper
- 1/4 teaspoon crushed red pepper flakes, optional
- 4 red snapper or orange roughy fillets (6 ounces each)

Directions:
1. In a large nonstick skillet coated with cooking spray, saute the zucchini, mushrooms and onion in 1 tablespoon oil until crisp-tender. Add the garlic; cook 1 minute longer. Stir in the tomatoes, basil, oregano, salt, pepper and, if desired, pepper flakes. Bring to a boil. Reduce heat; cover and simmer for 12-15 minutes or until vegetables are tender.
2. Meanwhile, in another large nonstick skillet coated with cooking spray, cook fillets in remaining oil over medium heat for 4-6 minutes on each side or until fish flakes easily with a fork. Serve with vegetable mixture.

61. Tuna With Citrus Ponzu Sauce

Servings: 4
Cooking Time: 20 Min
Ingredients:
- 1/2 teaspoon Chinese five-spice powder
- 1/4 teaspoon salt
- 1/4 teaspoon cayenne pepper
- 4 tuna steaks (6 ounces each)

- 1 tablespoon canola oil
- 1/4 cup orange juice
- 2 green onions, thinly sliced
- 1 tablespoon lemon juice
- 1 tablespoon reduced-sodium soy sauce
- 2 teaspoons rice vinegar
- 1 teaspoon brown sugar
- 1/4 teaspoon minced fresh gingerroot

Directions:
1. Combine the five-spice powder, salt and cayenne; sprinkle over tuna steaks. In a large skillet, cook tuna in oil over medium heat for 2-3 minutes on each side for medium-rare or until slightly pink in the center; remove and keep warm.
2. Combine the orange juice, onions, lemon juice, soy sauce, vinegar, brown sugar and ginger; pour into skillet. Cook for 1-2 minutes or until slightly thickened. Serve with tuna.

62. Tuna Cakes With Mustard Mayo

Servings: 4
Cooking Time: 30 Min
Ingredients:
- 2 large eggs
- 3 tablespoons minced fresh parsley, divided
- 1/2 teaspoon seafood seasoning
- 2 cans (5 ounces each) light water-packed tuna, drained and flaked
- 1/2 cup seasoned bread crumbs
- 1/2 cup shredded carrots
- 2 tablespoons butter, divided
- 1 package (12 ounces) frozen peas
- 1/4 teaspoon pepper
- 1/3 cup mayonnaise
- 1 tablespoon Dijon mustard
- 1 teaspoon 2% milk

Directions:
1. In a large bowl, combine the eggs, 2 tablespoons parsley and seafood seasoning. Stir in the tuna, bread crumbs and carrot. Shape into eight patties.
2. In a large skillet, brown patties in 1 tablespoon butter for 3-4 minutes on each side or until golden brown.
3. Meanwhile, microwave peas according to package directions. Stir in the pepper and remaining butter and parsley. Combine the mayonnaise, mustard and milk. Serve with tuna cakes and peas.

63. Spicy Tilapia Rice Bowl

Servings: 4
Cooking Time: 30 Min
Ingredients:
- 4 tilapia fillets (4 ounces each)
- 1 1/4 teaspoons Cajun seasoning
- 3 tablespoons olive oil, divided
- 1 medium yellow summer squash, halved lengthwise and sliced
- 1 package (16 ounces) frozen pepper and onion stir-fry blend
- 1 can (14 1/2 ounces) diced tomatoes, drained
- 1 envelope fajita seasoning mix
- 1 can (15 ounces) black beans, rinsed and drained
- 1/8 teaspoon salt
- 1/8 teaspoon pepper
- 3 cups hot cooked brown rice
- Optional toppings: cubed avocado, sour cream and salsa

Directions:

1.   Sprinkle fillets with Cajun seasoning. In a large skillet, heat 2 tablespoons oil over medium heat. Add fillets; cook 4-6 minutes on each side or until fish just begins to flake easily with a fork. Remove and keep warm. Wipe pan clean.

2.   In the same skillet, heat the remaining oil. Add squash; cook and stir 3 minutes. Add stir-fry blend and tomatoes; cook 6-8 minutes longer or until vegetables are tender. Stir in fajita seasoning mix; cook and stir 1-2 minutes longer or until slightly thickened.

3.   In a small bowl, mix beans, salt and pepper. Divide rice among four serving bowls; layer with beans, vegetables and fillets. Serve with toppings as desired.

64. Thai Lime Shrimp & Noodles

Servings: 6
Cooking Time: 25 Min
Ingredients:
- 1 cup minced fresh basil
- 3 tablespoons lime juice
- 4 teaspoons Thai red chili paste
- 1 garlic clove, minced
- 1 teaspoon minced fresh gingerroot
- 1 1/2 pounds uncooked shrimp (26-30 per pound), peeled and deveined
- 12 ounces cooked angel hair pasta
- 4 teaspoons olive oil, divided
- 1 can (14 1/2 ounces) chicken broth
- 1 can (13.66 ounces) coconut milk
- 1 teaspoon salt
- 1 tablespoon cornstarch
- 2 tablespoons cold water
- 2 tablespoons grated lime peel

Directions:

1.   Place the first five ingredients in a blender; cover and process until blended. Remove 1 tablespoon mixture; toss with shrimp.

2.   Cook pasta according to package directions. Meanwhile, in a large nonstick skillet, heat 2 teaspoons oil over medium-high heat. Add half of the shrimp mixture; stir-fry 2-4 minutes or until shrimp turn pink. Remove from pan; keep warm. Repeat with remaining oil and shrimp mixture.

3.   Add broth, coconut milk, salt and remaining basil mixture to same pan. In a small bowl, mix cornstarch and water until smooth. Stir into broth mixture. Bring to a boil; cook and stir 1-2 minutes or until slightly thickened. Stir in lime peel.

4.   Drain pasta; add pasta and shrimp to sauce, tossing to coat.

65. Honey And Citrus Salmon

Servings: 2
Cooking Time: 15 Minutes
Ingredients:
- 2 salmon fillets, skinned and deboned
- 1/6 cup of orange juice
- ¼ cup lemon juice
- 1-star anise piece
- ½ tsp honey
- ½ tbsp vegetable oil
- ½ tsp corn-flour
- Salt and pepper to taste

Directions:

1.   Combine the orange juice, lemon juice, star anise, and honey in a bowl. Season with salt and pepper and add the salmon fillets. Marinate in the fridge for 30 minutes.

2.   Heat oil in the skillet. Add the salmon fillets with some of the marinades. Cook for 3 minutes on each side.

3.   Add the remaining marinade after dissolving first in the corn-flour. Season with extra salt and pepper and cook for 2 minutes more. Serve.

66. Glazed Salmon Over Arugula Salad

Servings: 2
Cooking Time: 15 Minutes
Ingredients:
- ¼ cup maple syrup
- 1 ½ tbsps. lower-sodium soy sauce
- ½ tsp. Dijon mustard
- 1 tbsp. extra-virgin olive oil, divided
- 2 (5- to 6-ounce) salmon fillets
- ¼ cup chopped pecans
- 1 tbsp. apple cider vinegar
- 2 ounces baby arugula

Directions:
1.   Preheat the oven to 425F.
2.   In a bowl, stir together the maple syrup, soy sauce, and mustard.
3.   Heat half of the oil in a skillet. Add the salmon, skin-side down, and cook for 2 minutes or until the skin begins to brown.
4.   Spoon some of the sauce over each fillet. Reserve 2 tbsps. for the dressing and sprinkle the pecans over the fish.
5.   Transfer the skillet to the preheated oven and bake for 12 to 14 minutes, or until the fish is cooked.
6.   Meanwhile, add the apple cider vinegar and remaining oil to the reserved sauce mixture and whisk to mix. Toss the arugula with the dressing.
7.   Serve.

BEEF, PORK, AND LAMB

67. Merlot Filet Mignon

Servings: 2
Cooking Time: 20 Min
Ingredients:
- 2 beef tenderloin steaks (8 ounces each)
- 3 tablespoons butter, divided
- 1 tablespoon olive oil
- 1 cup merlot
- 2 tablespoons heavy whipping cream
- 1/8 teaspoon salt

Directions:
1. In a small skillet, cook steaks in 1 tablespoon butter and oil over medium heat for 4-6 minutes on each side or until meat reaches desired doneness (for medium-rare, a thermometer should read 145°; medium, 160°; well-done, 170°). Remove and keep warm.
2. In the same skillet, add wine, stirring to loosen browned bits from pan. Bring to a boil; cook until liquid is reduced to 1/4 cup. Add the cream, salt and remaining butter; bring to a boil. Cook and stir for 1-2 minutes or until slightly thickened and butter is melted. Serve with steaks.

68. Cashew Curried Beef

Servings: 5
Cooking Time: 20 Min
Ingredients:
- 1 pound beef top sirloin steak, thinly sliced
- 2 tablespoons canola oil, divided
- 1 can (13.66 ounces) coconut milk, divided
- 1 tablespoon red curry paste
- 2 tablespoons packed brown sugar
- 2 tablespoons fish sauce or soy sauce
- 8 cups chopped bok choy
- 1 small sweet red pepper, sliced
- 1/2 cup salted cashews
- 1/2 cup minced fresh cilantro
- Hot cooked brown rice

Directions:
1. In a large skillet, saute the beef in 1 tablespoon canola oil until no longer pink. Remove from skillet and set aside.
2. Spoon 1/2 cup cream from top of coconut milk and place in the pan. Add remaining oil; bring to a boil. Add curry paste; cook and stir for 5 minutes or until oil separates from coconut milk mixture.
3. Stir in the brown sugar, fish sauce and remaining coconut milk. Bring to a boil. Reduce heat; simmer, uncovered, 5 minutes or until slightly thickened. Add the chopped bok choy and red pepper; return to a boil. Cook and stir 2-3 minutes longer or until vegetables are tender.
4. Stir in the cashews, cilantro and beef; heat through. Serve with rice.

69. Oven-barbecued Pork Chops

Servings: 6-8
Cooking Time: 1 Hour
Ingredients:
- 6 to 8 loin or rib pork chops (3/4 inch thick)
- 1 tablespoon Worcestershire sauce
- 2 tablespoons vinegar
- 2 teaspoons brown sugar
- 1/2 teaspoon pepper

- 1/2 teaspoon chili powder
- 1/2 teaspoon paprika
- 3/4 cup ketchup
- 1/3 cup hot water

Directions:
1. Place chops in a heavy cast-iron skillet.
2. Combine all remaining ingredients; pour over chops. Bake, uncovered, at 375° for 1 hour.

70. Oven-roasted Ribs

Servings: 4
Cooking Time: 2 Hours 15 Minutes
Ingredients:
- 2¼ cups packed light brown sugar, divided
- 3 tablespoons chipotle powder, divided
- 2 tablespoons cayenne, plus 1 teaspoon
- 1 tablespoon garlic powder
- 1 tablespoon sea salt
- 1 teaspoon ground ginger
- 1 (1½- to 2-pound) rack of ribs, halved and patted dry
- 1 tablespoon olive oil
- 2 cups fresh Roma tomato puree or canned tomato puree
- Juice of 1 lemon

Directions:
1. Preheat the oven to 350°F.
2. In a small bowl, stir together 2 cups of brown sugar, 2 tablespoons of chipotle powder, 2 tablespoons of cayenne, the garlic powder, salt, and ginger. Rub the spice mixture into the ribs, coating all sides.
3. Heat the oil in the skillet over medium heat. Brown the ribs for 2 to 3 minutes per side. Turn off the heat.
4. Cover the skillet with a lid or aluminum foil and transfer it to the oven. Bake for 2 hours, or until the ribs are bubbling, browned, and the meat is falling off the bone.
5. When the ribs have about 20 minutes of cooking time left, in a small saucepan over low heat, combine the tomato puree and lemon juice, along with the remaining ¼ cup of brown sugar, 1 tablespoon of chipotle powder, and 1 teaspoon of cayenne. Simmer, stirring occasionally, until the ribs are done.
6. Remove the ribs from the oven, brush with the sauce, and return to the oven for 5 minutes. Brush the ribs a second time with sauce and let them rest for 5 minutes before serving.

71. The "perfect" Burger

Servings: 8-10 Servings
Cooking Time: 5 Minutes
Ingredients:
- 1 ½ pounds ground chuck
- 1 teaspoon coarse salt
- ½ teaspoon black pepper
- 1 white onion, sliced into rings
- 4 slices cheddar cheese (optional)
- 4 soft buns (such as potato buns), split

Directions:
1. Sprinkle ground beef with salt and pepper. Gently form the meat into 4 balls. Press the balls lightly into patties, 4-inches wide, 1-inch thick. Place an indentation in each burger's center with your thumb.
2. Place cast iron skillet on top of your outdoor grill and heat until it starts to smoke. Pour a small amount of vegetable oil into the skillet. Place burgers in skillet and lightly push down with a heavy duty spatula. After about 2-3 minutes, place sliced onion on top of burger. Flip burgers carefully so onions are on bottom and place a slice of cheese on alternate side. Cook 2 more minutes or until cheese melts. Serve burger on toasted bun, if desired.
Nutrition Info: Calories: 133, Sodium: 360 mg, Dietary Fiber: 0.7 g, Total Fat: 6.8 g, Total Carbs: 9.6 g, Protein: 8.0 g.

72. Prosciutto Pasta Toss

Servings: 6
Cooking Time: 20 Min
Ingredients:
- 1 package (16 ounces) linguine
- 1/2 cup frozen peas
- 2 tablespoons minced garlic
- 1 tablespoon Italian seasoning
- 1 teaspoon pepper
- 1/4 cup olive oil
- 1/2 pound thinly sliced prosciutto or deli ham, chopped
- 1/4 cup shredded Parmesan cheese

Directions:
1.   Cook linguine according to package directions, adding peas during the last 3 minutes.
2.   In a large skillet, saute the garlic, Italian seasoning and pepper in oil for 1 minute or until garlic is tender.
Stir in prosciutto. Drain linguine; add to the skillet and toss to coat. Sprinkle with cheese.

73. Bavarian Sausage Supper

Servings: 5
Cooking Time: 20 Min
Ingredients:
- 2 cups coleslaw mix
- 1 cup thinly sliced carrots
- 2 tablespoons butter
- 2 1/4 cups water
- 3/4 pound smoked kielbasa or Polish sausage, sliced into 1/4-inch pieces
- 1 package (4.9 ounces) quick-cooking noodles and sour cream and chive sauce mix
- 1/2 teaspoon caraway seeds, optional

Directions:
1.   In a large skillet, saute coleslaw mix and carrots in butter until crisp-tender. Add water; bring to a boil. Stir in the remaining ingredients. Return to a boil.
2.   Reduce heat; cover and cook for 8 minutes or until the noodles are tender, stirring occasionally.

74. Buttermilk Fried Chicken

Servings: 3-4 Servings
Cooking Time: 45 Minutes
Ingredients:
- 1 whole chicken (around 4 pounds), cut into pieces
- ½ carton buttermilk
- Salt
- ½ teaspoon cayenne pepper
- 1 ½ cups flour
- ½ tablespoon of each of the following: paprika, cumin, garlic powder, onion powder and celery salt
- Peanut oil for frying

Directions:
1.   Combine buttermilk, salt and cayenne pepper in a bowl. Several hours before frying chicken, marinate chicken in the buttermilk mixture in the refrigerator. Make sure chicken is evenly coated.
2.   Remove chicken from refrigerator and allow to reach room temperature. Combine flour with seasonings.
3.   Heat a cast iron skillet. Pour peanut oil in skillet until it comes up to about 1/3 of the skillet. With an instant read thermometer, the temperature of the oil should be about 350 degrees before frying the chicken.
4.   Remove the pieces of chicken from buttermilk mixture and shake dry. Dredge in flour. Repeat with remaining pieces. Once oil is hot enough, carefully place chicken in skillet. Keep an eye on the chicken and flip intermittently, making sure it does not burn. The thermometer inserted in the chicken should read about 165 degrees when chicken is fully cooked through.

5. Remove to a drying rack and liberally salt.
Nutrition Info: Calories: 868, Sodium: 293 mg, Dietary Fiber: 1.9 g, Total Fat: 14.5 g, Total Carbs: 38.2 g, Protein: 136.9 g.

75. Lamb Chops With Rosemary

Servings: 2
Cooking Time: 10 Minutes
Ingredients:
- 2 bone-in lamb chops, excess fat trimmed
- ½ small rosemary spring, chopped
- 1 ½ tbsps. olive oil
- 1 clove garlic
- 1 tbsp French mustard
- ½ tbsp vinegar
- Salt and pepper to taste

Directions:
1. Combine the rosemary, half of the oil, mustard, garlic, vinegar, and salt and pepper in a bowl.
2. Add the lamb chops to the bowl and coat well. Marinate in the fridge for 30 minutes.
3. Heat the remaining oil in the skillet and add the marinated pork chops.
4. Cook for 4 minutes on each side. Serve.

76. Sloppy Joes

Servings: 4
Cooking Time: 25 Minutes
Ingredients:
- 1 tablespoon salted butter
- 1 pound ground beef, 85% lean
- ½ yellow onion, diced
- 3 garlic cloves, minced
- ¾ cup ketchup
- 8 ounces crushed tomatoes
- ¼ teaspoon sea salt
- 2 tablespoons hot sauce
- 1 tablespoon Worcestershire sauce
- ½ tablespoon brown sugar
- 1 tablespoon spicy brown mustard
- 1 teaspoon smoked paprika
- ¼ teaspoon red pepper flakes
- 4 hamburger buns

Directions:
1. In your skillet, melt the butter over medium-high heat. Add the ground beef to the pan and stir to break up.
2. Cook for 3 to 4 minutes until browned. Add the onion and garlic, stir, and continue to cook.
3. In a medium bowl, whisk together the ketchup, tomatoes, salt, hot sauce, Worcestershire sauce, sugar, mustard, paprika, and red pepper flakes.
4. Add the tomato mixture to the skillet, stirring well to coat the beef.
5. Once the pan is bubbling, cover and reduce the heat, simmering for 12 to 15 minutes.
6. Remove the cover and stir. Season to taste.
7. Scoop a generous amount onto each bun and serve hot.

77. Contest-winning German Pizza

Servings: 4-6
Cooking Time: 40 Min
Ingredients:

- 1 pound ground beef
- 1/2 medium onion, chopped
- 1/2 green pepper, diced
- 1 1/2 teaspoon salt, divided
- 1/2 teaspoon pepper
- 2 tablespoons butter
- 6 medium potatoes (about 2 1/4 pounds), peeled and finely shredded
- 3 large eggs, lightly beaten
- 1/3 cup milk
- 2 cups (8 ounces) shredded cheddar or part-skim mozzarella cheese

Directions:
1. In a large skillet over medium heat, cook and stir ground beef, onion, green pepper, 1/2 teaspoon salt and pepper until meat is no longer pink; drain. Remove and keep warm.
2. Reduce heat to low; melt butter in pan. Spread potatoes over butter and sprinkle with remaining salt. Top with beef mixture. Combine eggs and milk; pour over all.
3. Cover and cook 30 minutes or until set in the center. Sprinkle with mozzarella cheese; cover and cook until cheese is melted. Cut into wedges.

78. Skillet Pork Chops With Zucchini

Servings: 6
Cooking Time: 35 Min
Ingredients:
- 3 tablespoons all-purpose flour
- 2 tablespoons plus 1/4 cup grated Parmesan cheese, divided
- 1 1/2 teaspoons salt
- 1/2 teaspoon dill weed
- 1/4 teaspoon pepper
- 6 boneless pork loin chops (4 ounces each)
- 1 tablespoon canola oil
- 2 medium onions, sliced
- 1/4 cup warm water
- 3 medium zucchini (about 1 pound), sliced
- 1/2 teaspoon paprika

Directions:
1. In a shallow dish, combine the flour, 2 tablespoons cheese, salt, dill and pepper. Dip pork chops in the flour mixture to coat both sides; shake off excess.
2. In a large skillet, brown chops on both sides in oil. Top with the onions; add water. Bring to a boil. Reduce heat; cover and simmer for 15 minutes.
3. Place the zucchini over the onions. Sprinkle the remaining cheese over zucchini. Sprinkle with paprika. Cover and simmer for 10-15 minutes or until the vegetables are tender and a thermometer inserted in pork reads 145°. Let stand 5 minutes.

79. Skillet Chicken Sausage And Red Beans

Servings: 2-4 Servings
Cooking Time: 15 Minutes
Ingredients:
- 1 tablespoon olive oil
- ½ pound spicy chicken sausage
- 1 onion, sliced thin
- 3 garlic cloves, minced
- 1 teaspoon creole seasoning
- ½ cup chicken or vegetable stock
- 15 ounce can kidney beans, drained and rinsed
- 2 tablespoons flat fresh leaf parsley

Directions:

1. Heat olive oil in cast iron skillet and break up sausage in skillet, sautéing until browned, 3-4 minutes.
2. Add onion and sauté until softened, 4 minutes. Add garlic and seasoning and stir. Add the stock and cover the pan, cooking 2 minutes.
3. Uncover, add the beans and sausage and cook another five minutes. Take skillet off the heat. Sprinkle with parsley.
Nutrition Info: Calories: 183, Sodium: 655 mg, Dietary Fiber: 6.4 g, Total Fat: 5.8 g, Total Carbs: 19.8 g, Protein: 13.9 g.

80. Muffuletta Pasta

Servings: 8
Cooking Time: 25 Min
Ingredients:
- 1 package (16 ounces) bow tie pasta
- 1 bunch green onions, chopped
- 2 teaspoons plus 1/4 cup butter, divided
- 1 tablespoon minced garlic
- 1 package (16 ounces) cubed fully cooked ham
- 1 jar (12.36 ounces) tapenade or ripe olive bruschetta topping, drained
- 1 package (3 1/2 ounces) sliced pepperoni
- 1 cup heavy whipping cream
- 2 cups (8 ounces) shredded Italian cheese blend

Directions:
1. Cook pasta according to package directions. Meanwhile, in a large skillet, saute the onions in 2 teaspoons butter until tender. Add garlic; cook for 1 minute longer. Add the ham, tapenade and pepperoni; saute 2 minutes longer.
2. Cube remaining butter; stir butter and cream into the skillet. Bring to a boil over medium heat. Reduce heat; simmer, uncovered, for 3 minutes.
3. Drain pasta; toss with ham mixture. Sprinkle with cheese.

81. Sweet And Sticky Short Ribs

Servings: 6 Servings
Cooking Time: 4 Hours And 15 Minutes
Ingredients:
- 3 pounds shirt ribs, English cut
- ½ cup soy sauce
- 1 cup light brown sugar
- ¼ cup Thai sweet chili sauce
- 5 garlic cloves, smashed
- Salt and black pepper, to taste
- 1 inch piece of grated ginger
- ½ cup beef broth
- ½ cup water

Directions:
1. Preheat oven to 300 degrees.
2. Combine soy sauce, brown sugar, sweet chili sauce, garlic, salt, pepper and ginger in a bowl. Place ribs in marinade for 1-2 hours in the refrigerator. Remove ribs and reserve marinade. Pat dry.
3. Heat a cast iron Dutch oven over medium heat. Place ribs in pot but don't crowd the vessel. Sear on all sides, 3-4 minutes per side. Brown the ribs in rotation if necessary. Place all ribs back in pot. Mix the reserved marinade with the water and broth and pour into the Dutch oven. Cover with lid and cook in oven for 3-4 hours, or until meat is falling off the bone.
4. When ribs are done, refrigerate them with the sauce. After fat has been skimmed, you can pour sauce into pot and heat to reduce it slightly.
Nutrition Info: Calories: 130, Sodium: 1339 mg, Dietary Fiber: 0 g, Total Fat: 0.1 g, Total Carbs: 30.9 g, Protein: 1.9 g.

82. Chili Beef Noodle Skillet

Servings: 8
Cooking Time: 30 Min
Ingredients:
- 1 package (8 ounces) egg noodles
- 2 pounds ground beef
- 1 medium onion, chopped
- 1/4 cup chopped celery
- 2 garlic cloves, minced
- 1 can (28 ounces) diced tomatoes, undrained
- 1 tablespoon chili powder
- 1/4 to 1/2 teaspoon salt
- 1/8 teaspoon pepper
- 1/2 to 1 cup shredded cheddar cheese

Directions:
1.   Cook noodles according to package directions. Meanwhile, in a large skillet, cook the beef, onion, celery and garlic over medium heat until meat is no longer pink and vegetables are tender; drain. Add the tomatoes, chili powder, salt and pepper. Cook and stir for 2 minutes or until heated through.
2.   Drain the noodles; stir into beef mixture and heat through. Remove from the heat. Sprinkle with cheddar cheese; cover and let stand for 5 minutes or until cheese is melted.

83.   Saucy Beef & Broccoli

Servings: 2
Cooking Time: 30 Min
Ingredients:
- 1 tablespoon cornstarch
- 1/2 cup water
- 1/2 teaspoon beef stock concentrate
- 1/4 cup sherry or additional beef broth
- 2 tablespoons reduced-sodium soy sauce
- 1 tablespoon brown sugar
- 1 garlic clove, minced
- 1 teaspoon minced fresh gingerroot
- 2 teaspoons canola oil, divided
- 1/2 pound beef top sirloin steak, cut into 1/4-inch strips
- 2 cups fresh broccoli florets
- 8 green onions, cut into 1-inch pieces

Directions:
1.   In a small bowl, mix the first eight ingredients. In a large nonstick skillet, heat 1 teaspoon oil over medium-high heat. Add beef; stir-fry 1-2 minutes or until no longer pink. Remove from pan.
2.   Stir-fry broccoli in remaining oil 4-5 minutes or until crisp-tender. Add green onions; cook 1-2 minutes longer or just until tender.
3.   Stir cornstarch mixture and add to pan. Bring to a boil; cook and stir for 2-3 minutes or until thickened. Return beef to pan; heat through.

84.   Beef Stew Skillet Pie

Servings: 4 To 6
Cooking Time: 1 Hour
Ingredients:
- FOR THE DOUGH
- 1¼ cups all-purpose flour
- 1 teaspoon paprika
- ¼ teaspoon salt
- 1½ sticks cold butter, cubed

- 2 to 4 tablespoons cold water
- 1 egg
- FOR THE FILLING
- 1 tablespoon olive oil
- 1 pound stew beef, cubed
- 1 tablespoon salted butter
- 1 leek, thinly sliced
- 5 red potatoes, quartered
- 1 large carrot, cut into ½" rounds
- 1 onion, minced
- 4 garlic cloves, minced
- 1 teaspoon ground ginger
- 1 tablespoon Worcestershire sauce
- 2 tablespoons all-purpose flour
- 1 teaspoon sea salt
- ½ cup red wine
- 2 cups beef broth

Directions:
1. In a large bowl, combine the flour, paprika, salt, and butter. Use your hands to cut the butter in, until the texture resembles cornmeal. Pour in the water, a little at a time, until a dough ball forms. Wrap the dough in plastic wrap and chill for 20 to 30 minutes.
2. In your skillet, heat the oil over medium heat. Add the beef and brown on all sides, 4 to 5 minutes, and then remove to a plate.
3. Add the butter to the hot skillet. Once it begins to melt, add the leek, potatoes, carrots, onion, and garlic. Cook for 4 to 5 minutes, stirring frequently, until tender and brown around the edges.
4. Stir in the ginger, Worcestershire sauce, flour, and salt. Stir to coat, then add the red wine. Add the beef broth to the pan and stir to combine. Reduce the heat and simmer for 10 to 15 minutes, stirring occasionally.
5. Heat the oven to 400°F.
6. While the meat is simmering, roll out the dough onto a floured surface. Shape it into a 13" round.
7. Remove the skillet from the heat and stir the stew well to redistribute the liquid. Place the pie dough on top, pressing it in around the edges of the skillet. Cut 4 slits from the center toward the edges, about 3" in length.
8. Whisk the egg in a small bowl, then brush over the top of the dough.
9. Bake the pie for 25 to 30 minutes, until the crust is golden brown. Serve warm.

85. Lamb Chops With Herb Butter

Servings: 2
Cooking Time: 15 Minutes
Ingredients:
- 4 lamb chops
- Sea salt
- 1 teaspoon fresh thyme leaves, minced, plus 1 tablespoon
- 6 tablespoons salted butter, room temperature, divided
- 1 tablespoon fresh rosemary leaves, minced
- 1 tablespoon fresh oregano leaves, minced
- 2 garlic cloves, minced

Directions:
1. Season the lamb chops with salt to taste and 1 teaspoon of thyme. Let the lamb rest while you make the herb butter.
2. In a small bowl, thoroughly combine 4 tablespoons of butter, the remaining 1 tablespoon of thyme, the rosemary, oregano, and garlic.
3. In the skillet over medium-high heat, melt the remaining 2 tablespoons of butter. Cook the lamb for 5 to 6 minutes, flip, and cook it for 5 to 6 minutes more, or until the internal temperature reaches 145°F. Let the lamb rest for 5 minutes.
4. Serve each chop with a dollop of herb butter on top.

86. Parmesan Pork Cutlets

Servings: 4
Cooking Time: 15 Min
Ingredients:
- 1 pork tenderloin (1 pound)
- 1/3 cup all-purpose flour
- 2 large eggs, lightly beaten
- 1 cup dry bread crumbs
- 1/4 cup grated Parmesan cheese
- 1 teaspoon salt
- 1/4 cup olive oil
- Lemon wedges

Directions:
1.   Cut pork diagonally into eight slices; pound each to 1/4-in. thickness. Place flour and eggs in separate shallow bowls. In another shallow bowl, combine the bread crumbs, cheese and salt. Dip pork in the flour, eggs, then bread crumb mixture.
2.   In a large skillet, cook pork in oil in batches over medium heat for 2-3 minutes on each side or until crisp and the meat juices run clear. Remove and keep warm. Serve with lemon wedges.

87. Cabbage Roll Skillet

Servings: 6
Cooking Time: 20 Min
Ingredients:
- 1 can (28 ounces) whole plum tomatoes, undrained
- 1 pound extra-lean ground beef (95% lean)
- 1 large onion, chopped
- 1 can (8 ounces) tomato sauce
- 2 tablespoons cider vinegar
- 1 tablespoon brown sugar
- 1 teaspoon dried oregano
- 1 teaspoon dried thyme
- 1/2 teaspoon pepper
- 1 small head cabbage, thinly sliced (about 6 cups)
- 1 medium green pepper, cut into thin strips
- 4 cups hot cooked brown rice

Directions:
1.   Drain the plum tomatoes, reserving liquid; coarsely chop tomatoes. In a large nonstick skillet, cook beef and onion over medium-high heat for 6-8 minutes or until the beef is no longer pink, breaking up beef into crumbles. Stir in tomato sauce, vinegar, brown sugar, seasonings and the tomatoes and reserved liquid.
2.   Add cabbage and green pepper; cook, covered, 6 minutes, stirring occasionally. Cook, uncovered, 6-8 minutes longer or until cabbage is tender. Serve with rice.

88. Marvelous Meatloaf

Servings: 2
Cooking Time: 40 Minutes
Ingredients:
- 1-pound ground beef
- 1 egg
- 18 butter crackers, crushed
- ½ tbsp. seasoning salt
- ¼ white onion, finely chopped
- ½ tbsp. Worcestershire sauce
- ¼ tsp. freshly ground black pepper
- 1 tbsp. olive oil

- 2 tbsps. ketchup

Directions:
1. In a bowl, mix the ground beef, eggs, crackers, seasoning salt, onion, Worcestershire sauce, and pepper. Shape into a round loaf.
2. Heat oil in the skillet.
3. Add the meatloaf and sear each side for 3 to 5 minutes. Brush the ketchup over the top and cover. Move to low heat.
4. Cook, covered, for 20 to 30 minutes or until the meat is cooked through.
5. Remove from the heat and sit for 5 to 10 minutes. Drain any excess liquid and serve.

89. Dry-rubbed Pork Chops

Servings: 2
Cooking Time: 30 Minutes
Ingredients:
- 2 bone-in, center-cut pork chops
- 1 tsp. oil
- ¼ tsp. cumin
- ¼ tsp. coriander
- ¼ tsp. brown sugar
- ¼ tsp. black pepper
- ¼ tsp. salt

Directions:
1. Preheat the oven to 400F. Preheat the skillet.
2. Rub pork chops with oil. Combine the remainder of spices and sprinkle on chops.
3. Cook pork chops in the skillet and cook 3 minutes per side.
4. Then transfer the pan with the chops to the oven and cook until the chops reach 140 to 145F. Start checking the chops after 5 minutes, then check every minute thereafter. This should take about 10 minutes.
5. Remove the chops and rest for 10 to 15 minutes. Serve.

90. Tuscan Lamb Chops

Servings: 2
Cooking Time: 15 Minutes
Ingredients:
- 2 tsps. minced garlic
- 1 tsp. Dijon mustard
- 4 tbsps. olive oil, divided
- 1 tsp. minced fresh thyme
- 2 tsps. minced fresh rosemary
- ½ tsp. Kosher salt, plus more
- ½ tsp. black pepper, plus more
- 1.25 pounds lamb loin chops (1 ½-2 inch thick)
- 1 tbsp. butter

Directions:
1. In a bowl, combine mustard, garlic, 3 tbsps. oil, herbs, and ½ tsp. each of salt and pepper.
2. Add the lamb chops and coat well. Cover and marinate in the refrigerator for about 8 hours. Flip once. Remove the chops 30 minutes before cooking.
3. Preheat the oven to 425F.
4. Pat dry the chops with a paper towel. Then season with salt and pepper.
5. Preheat the cast-iron skillet. Add butter and remaining oil.
6. Sear the lamb chops 2 minutes per side.
7. Transfer the skillet to the oven and cook for 4 to 6 minutes for medium-rare.
8. Remove from the oven and cover with a foil. Rest for 10 minutes and serve.

91. Seared Short Ribs With Lime Cabbage Slaw

Servings: 4
Cooking Time: 10 Minutes
Ingredients:
- For the lime cabbage slaw
- 2 cups shredded green cabbage
- 2 cups shredded red cabbage
- ½ red onion, thinly sliced
- 2 garlic cloves, minced
- ½ teaspoon sea salt
- 1 tablespoon mayonnaise
- Juice of 2 limes
- 2 tablespoons fresh cilantro
- For the short ribs
- 2 tablespoons olive oil
- 1 pound boneless beef short ribs, 1-inch thick, at room temperature
- Pinch sea salt
- Pinch freshly ground black pepper

Directions:
1.   To make the lime cabbage slaw: In a medium bowl, combine the green and red cabbage, onion, garlic, salt, mayonnaise, lime juice, and cilantro. Mix thoroughly and chill in the refrigerator.
2.   To make the short ribs: Heat the oil in the skillet over medium-high heat.
3.   Season the ribs with salt and pepper.
4.   Cook the ribs for 3 to 4 minutes per side, or until nicely browned. Let them rest for 5 minutes.
5.   Thinly slice the ribs and serve with the slaw.

92. One-pan Chicken Enchiladas

Servings: 6-8 Servings
Cooking Time: 1 Hour
Ingredients:
- 1 tablespoon olive oil
- 1 onion chopped
- 1 cup frozen corn
- 3 canned chipotle chiles, seeded and minced
- 1 (28 ounce) can stewed tomatoes
- 3 cups cooked and shredded chicken (roasted, poached etc.)
- 12 corn tortillas
- Enchilada sauce (canned)
- 1 ½ cups combination of shredded pepper jack and cheddar cheeses
- Cilantro leaves, chopped scallions, sour cream for garnish

Directions:
1.   Preheat oven to 375 degrees.
2.   Heat cast iron skillet over medium heat. Sauté onion in olive oil. Add corn, chiles and stewed tomatoes and stir. Add shredded chicken and coat thoroughly.
3.   Place chicken on a plate. Wipe out skillet. Spoon about 1/3 of the enchilada sauce on the bottom of the skillet. Spoon chicken mixture into each of the tortillas. Roll tortillas and place seam side down in the skillet. Repeat until skillet is full. Pour remaining enchilada sauce over tortillas and top with cheese.
4.   Bake in oven for about 25 minutes. Top with cilantro, scallions and sour cream.
Nutrition Info: Calories: 1832, Sodium: 2909 mg, Dietary Fiber: 4.6 g, Total Fat: 135.5 g, Total Carbs: 46.0 g, Protein: 110.4 g.

93. Rosemary Roasted Veal Chops

Servings: 2 Servings
Cooking Time: 30 Minutes

Ingredients:
- 2 veal chops
- Coarse salt
- Black pepper
- 2 tablespoons olive oil
- 4 garlic cloves, minced
- 2 sprigs rosemary, minced
- Lemon wedges

Directions:
1. Remove veal chops from refrigerator and allow to come to room temperature. Preheat a cast iron skillet over medium heat. Preheat oven to 375 degrees.
2. Sprinkle chops with salt and pepper. Once skillet is hot, add olive oil. Place chops in skillet, making sure not to overcrowd the skillet.
3. Sear on all sides until golden brown, about 3-4 minutes. Remove chop from pan and sprinkle with garlic and rosemary mixture. Place chop in oven and roast for 8-10 minutes, turning once.
4. Remove veal chops and allow to rest for 10 minutes. Serve with lemon on the side.

Nutrition Info: Calories: 723, Sodium: 1801 mg, Dietary Fiber: 0 g, Total Fat: 9.3 g, Total Carbs: 4.0 g, Protein: 0.2 g.

94. Beef & Spinach Lo Mein

Servings: 5
Cooking Time: 30 Min
Ingredients:
- 1/4 cup hoisin sauce
- 2 tablespoons soy sauce
- 1 tablespoon water
- 2 teaspoons sesame oil
- 2 garlic cloves, minced
- 1/4 teaspoon crushed red pepper flakes
- 1 pound beef top round steak, thinly sliced
- 6 ounces uncooked spaghetti
- 4 teaspoons canola oil, divided
- 1 can (8 ounces) sliced water chestnuts, drained
- 2 green onions, sliced
- 1 package (10 ounces) fresh spinach, coarsely chopped
- 1 red chili pepper, seeded and thinly sliced

Directions:
1. In a small bowl, mix the first six ingredients. Remove 1/4 cup mixture to a large bowl; add beef and toss to coat. Marinate at room temperature 10 minutes.
2. Cook spaghetti according to package directions. Meanwhile, in a large skillet, heat 1 1/2 teaspoons canola oil. Add half of the beef mixture; stir-fry 1-2 minutes or until no longer pink. Remove from pan. Repeat with an additional 1 1/2 teaspoons oil and remaining beef mixture.
3. Stir-fry water chestnuts and green onions in remaining canola oil 30 seconds. Stir in spinach and remaining hoisin mixture; cook until spinach is wilted. Return beef to pan; heat through.
4. Drain spaghetti; add to beef mixture and toss to combine. Sprinkle with chili pepper.

95. Blt Skillet

Servings: 2
Cooking Time: 25 Min
Ingredients:
- 4 ounces uncooked whole wheat linguine
- 4 bacon strips, cut into 1 1/2-inch pieces
- 1 plum tomato, cut into 1-inch pieces
- 1 garlic clove, minced
- 1 1/2 teaspoons lemon juice

- 1/4 teaspoon salt
- 1/4 teaspoon pepper
- 2 tablespoons grated Parmesan cheese
- 1 tablespoon minced fresh parsley

Directions:

1. Cook linguine according to package directions. Meanwhile, in a large skillet, cook the bacon over medium heat until crisp. Remove to paper towels; drain, reserving 1 teaspoon drippings.
2. In the drippings, saute the tomato and garlic for 1-2 minutes or until heated through. Stir in the bacon, lemon juice, salt and pepper.
3. Drain the linguine; add to the skillet. Sprinkle with cheese and parsley; toss to coat.

96. Bacon-swiss Pork Chops

Servings: 4
Cooking Time: 25 Min
Ingredients:

- 2 bacon strips, chopped
- 1 medium onion, chopped
- 4 boneless pork loin chops (4 ounces each)
- 1/2 teaspoon garlic powder
- 1/4 teaspoon salt
- 2 slices reduced-fat Swiss cheese, halved

Directions:

1. In a nonstick skillet coated with cooking spray, cook bacon and onion over medium heat until the bacon is crisp, stirring occasionally. Drain on paper towels; discard drippings.
2. Sprinkle the pork chops with garlic powder and salt. Add pork chops to the same pan; cook over medium heat for 3-4 minutes on each side or until a thermometer reads 145°. Top the pork with the bacon mixture and cheese. Cook, covered, on low heat 1-2 minutes or until the cheese is melted. Let stand 5 minutes before serving.

97. Stewed Lamb With Cilantro And Mint

Servings: 2
Cooking Time: 1 Hour And 20 Minutes
Ingredients:

- 1 ½ tbsps. butter
- 1-pound lamb cut into 1-inch cubes
- ½ large onion, chopped
- 2 Roma tomatoes, cubed
- 1 ½ tbsp. tomato paste
- 1 plum, pitted and chopped
- 1 ½ cups broth
- ½ tbsp. chopped dill
- ½ tbsp. chopped cilantro
- 1 tbsp. chopped mint
- Juice of ½ lemon
- Salt and pepper to taste

Directions:

1. Melt the butter in the skillet. Add the lamb and cook for 10 minutes or until browned on all sides.
2. Remove the meat from the skillet and add the onion. Cook for 8 to 10 minutes. Add the tomatoes, tomato paste, and plums. Mix well.
3. Stir in the chicken broth and the herbs. Add the lamb to the skillet, and cover.
4. Lower heat to low and simmer for 1 hour or until the lamb is cooked.
5. Stir in the lemon juice and season with salt and pepper. Serve.

98. Braised Beef In Wine Sauce

Servings: 6-10 Servings
Cooking Time: 3 Hours And 30 Minutes
Ingredients:
- 2 tablespoons butter
- 2 tablespoons olive oil
- 5 pound beef chuck roast
- Coarse salt and freshly ground pepper
- 2 Vidalia onions, cut into 1/8ths
- 4 cloves garlic, minced
- 4 carrots, quartered
- 2 medium potatoes, quartered
- 2 cup good quality dry red wine
- 1 bouquet garni, containing 2 sprigs thyme, 1 bay leaf, I bunch parsley, 1 sprig oregano, tied with a string

Directions:
1.   Preheat the oven to 300 degrees. Preheat an enameled cast iron casserole pan or Dutch oven over medium heat.
2.   Melt butter and olive oil. Dry meat thoroughly and sprinkle generously with salt and pepper. Place meat in pan and sear until brown on each side, about 4 minutes. Press down lightly with a rubber spatula. Transfer meat to a dish.
3.   Add onions, garlic, carrots and potatoes and stir vegetables, scraping up brown bits from bottom until softened, 6-8 minutes. Pour in wine. Add bouquet garni and additional salt. Turn up heat to medium-high and cook for 10-15 minutes until liquid reduces. Place meat inside Dutch oven and cover tightly. Place in oven and cook for 3 hours or longer until meat is very tender. Check meat periodically to ensure that the liquid has not evaporated.

Nutrition Info: Calories: 958, Sodium: 184 mg, Dietary Fiber: 2.1 g, Total Fat: 68.3 g, Total Carbs: 12.8 g, Protein: 60.6 g.

99. Chuck Wagon Tortilla Stack

Servings: 4-6
Cooking Time: 40 Min
Ingredients:
- 1 pound ground beef
- 2 to 3 garlic cloves, minced
- 1 can (16 ounces) baked beans
- 1 can (14 1/2 ounces) stewed tomatoes, undrained
- 1 can (11 ounces) whole kernel corn, drained
- 1 can (4 ounces) chopped green chilies
- 1/4 cup barbecue sauce
- 4 1/2 teaspoons chili powder
- 1 1/2 teaspoons ground cumin
- 4 flour tortillas (10 inches)
- 1 1/3 cups (about 5 ounces) shredded pepper jack cheese
- Shredded lettuce, chopped red onion, sour cream and/or chopped tomatoes, optional

Directions:
1.   In a large skillet, cook beef until no longer pink; drain. Add garlic, beans, tomatoes, corn, chilies, barbecue sauce, chili powder and cumin. Bring to a boil. Reduce heat; simmer, uncovered, for 10-12 minutes or until liquid is reduced.
2.   Coat a large deep skillet with cooking spray. Place one tortilla in skillet; spread with 1 1/2 cups meat mixture. Sprinkle with 1/3 cup cheese. Repeat layers three times. Cover and cook on low for 15 minutes or until cheese is melted and tortillas are heated through. Cut into wedges. Serve with toppings of your choice.

VEGAN & VEGETARIAN

100.Zucchini Burgers

Servings: 4
Cooking Time: 5 Min/batch
Ingredients:
- 2 cups shredded zucchini
- 1 medium onion, finely chopped
- 1/2 cup dry bread crumbs
- 2 large eggs, lightly beaten
- 1/8 teaspoon salt
- Dash cayenne pepper
- 3 hard-cooked large egg whites, chopped
- 2 tablespoons canola oil
- 4 whole wheat hamburger buns, split
- 4 lettuce leaves
- 4 slices tomato
- 4 slices onion

Directions:
1. In a sieve or colander, drain zucchini, squeezing to remove excess liquid. Pat dry. In a small bowl, combine the zucchini, onion, bread crumbs, eggs, salt and cayenne. Gently stir in cooked egg whites.
2. Heat 1 tablespoon oil in a large nonstick skillet over medium-low heat. Drop the mixture by scant 2/3 cupfuls into the oil; press lightly to flatten. Fry in batches until patties are golden brown on both sides, using remaining oil as needed.
3. Serve on buns with lettuce, tomato and onion.

101.Curried Tofu With Rice

Servings: 4
Cooking Time: 20 Min
Ingredients:
- 1 package (12.3 ounces) extra-firm tofu, drained and cubed
- 1 teaspoon seasoned salt
- 1 tablespoon canola oil
- 1 small onion, chopped
- 3 garlic cloves, minced
- 1/2 cup light coconut milk
- 1/4 cup minced fresh cilantro
- 1 teaspoon curry powder
- 1/4 teaspoon salt
- 1/4 teaspoon pepper
- 2 cups cooked brown rice

Directions:
1. Sprinkle tofu with the seasoned salt. In a large nonstick skillet coated with cooking spray, saute the tofu in oil until lightly browned. Remove and keep warm.
2. In the same skillet, saute the onion and garlic for 1-2 minutes or until crisp-tender. Stir in the coconut milk, cilantro, curry, salt and pepper. Bring to a boil. Reduce heat; simmer, uncovered, 4-5 minutes or until sauce is slightly thickened. Stir in tofu; heat through. Serve with rice.

102.Eggplant Lasagna

Servings: 4 To 6
Cooking Time: 1 Hour 20 Minutes
Ingredients:
- 2 tablespoons olive oil
- 1 white onion, chopped

- 4 garlic cloves, minced
- 1 (6-ounce) can tomato paste
- 1 (28-ounce) can diced tomatoes
- ½ cup water
- 1 teaspoon sea salt, divided
- 2 cups ricotta
- 1 large egg
- 1 tablespoon dried oregano, divided
- ½ teaspoon freshly ground black pepper, divided
- 1 pound dried lasagna noodles, divided
- 1 large eggplant, thinly sliced into rounds, divided
- 8 ounces fresh mozzarella cheese, cut into ¼-inch slices, divided
- ¼ teaspoon red pepper flakes
- 1 cup grated Parmesan cheese

Directions:
1. Heat the oil in the skillet over medium heat.
2. Add the onion and garlic and cook for 3 to 5 minutes, stirring frequently, until the onion is translucent.
3. Add the tomato paste and mix well. Smear the paste around the skillet to brown it and cook for 1 to 2 minutes. Add the diced tomatoes with their juices and stir until the tomato paste and tomatoes are well combined. Add the water and ¼ teaspoon of salt. Reduce the heat to low and simmer for 20 to 25 minutes.
4. Remove the skillet from the heat and transfer two-thirds of the sauce to a bowl.
5. Preheat the oven to 400°F.
6. In a small bowl, whisk the ricotta, egg, 1½ teaspoons of oregano, ½ teaspoon of salt, and ¼ teaspoon of pepper to combine.
7. Place a layer of dried noodles into the sauce in the skillet. Top the noodles with half the ricotta mixture, a layer of eggplant, then about a quarter of the remaining sauce.
8. Add a second layer of noodles. Top it with half of the mozzarella cheese and another quarter of the remaining sauce.
9. Add a third layer of noodles. Top it with the rest of the ricotta mixture, another layer of eggplant, and about half the remaining sauce.
10. Add a final layer of noodles. Top it with the remaining sauce, then finish with the remaining half of the mozzarella cheese, the Parmesan cheese, and the remaining ¼ teaspoon of salt, ¼ teaspoon of black pepper, and 1½ teaspoons of oregano.
11. Lightly cover the skillet with aluminum foil. Bake for 30 to 35 minutes. Remove the foil and bake, uncovered, for 10 minutes more, or until the cheese is melted and bubbling.

103.Macaroni And Cheese

Servings: 4 To 6
Cooking Time: 40 To 45 Minutes
Ingredients:
- 1 pound dry macaroni
- 6 ounces fresh mozzarella cheese, cubed
- 1 tablespoon olive oil
- 1 cup whole milk
- 1 cup heavy cream
- 2 garlic cloves, minced
- 4 tablespoons salted butter
- 2 tablespoons all-purpose flour
- 1 cup shredded Swiss cheese
- Juice of 1 lemon
- 1 teaspoon sea salt, plus more for seasoning
- 1 teaspoon cayenne
- 1 cup shredded Parmesan cheese

Directions:
1. Preheat the oven to 350°F.
2. In a medium pot, cook the macaroni according to the package directions. Drain the pasta and return it to the pot. Add the mozzarella and olive oil to the pot and stir well.

3. In a small saucepan, scald the milk, cream, and garlic. Remove from the heat and set aside.
4. Melt the butter in your skillet over medium heat. Slowly whisk the flour into the butter, continuing to whisk for 1 to 2 minutes until it begins to thicken and smooth out. Pour the milk mixture in, a little at a time, and whisk quickly to prevent clumping.
5. Add the Swiss cheese to the sauce, whisking constantly until the cheese melts. Remove the pan from the heat and add the lemon juice and salt.
6. Stir the pasta into the cheese sauce, mixing well to coat all the macaroni. Sprinkle with the cayenne and salt. Top with the Parmesan cheese.
7. Bake for 35 to 40 minutes, until browned and bubbling.

104.Skillet Pasta Florentine

Servings: 6
Cooking Time: 35 Min
Ingredients:
- 3 cups uncooked spiral pasta
- 1 large egg, lightly beaten
- 2 cups (16 ounces) 2% cottage cheese
- 1 1/2 cups reduced-fat ricotta cheese
- 1 package (10 ounces) frozen chopped spinach, thawed and squeezed dry
- 1 cup (4 ounces) shredded part-skim mozzarella cheese, divided
- 1 teaspoon each dried parsley flakes, oregano and basil
- 1 jar (14 ounces) meatless spaghetti sauce
- 2 tablespoons grated Parmesan cheese

Directions:
1. Cook pasta according to package directions. Meanwhile, in a large bowl, combine the egg, cottage cheese, ricotta, spinach, 1/2 cup of the mozzarella and herbs.
2. Drain pasta. Place half of the sauce in a large skillet; layer with pasta and remaining sauce. Top with cheese mixture.
3. Bring to a boil. Reduce heat; cover and cook for 25-30 minutes or until a thermometer reads 160°.
4. Sprinkle with Parmesan cheese and remaining mozzarella cheese; cover and cook for 5 minutes longer or until the cheese is melted. Let stand for 5 minutes before serving.

105.Curried Pea And Mushroom Shepherd's Pie

Servings: 4 To 6
Cooking Time: 1 Hour 10 Minutes
Ingredients:
- For the potatoes
- 3 russet potatoes, peeled and quartered
- 8 tablespoons (1 stick) salted butter
- ½ cup mayonnaise
- 1 teaspoon sea salt, plus more as needed
- 1 teaspoon cumin seed
- 1 teaspoon fennel seed
- 1 teaspoon ground coriander
- 1 teaspoon curry powder
- ½ teaspoon garam masala
- ½ teaspoon cayenne
- For the filling
- 2 tablespoons salted butter
- 1 white onion, minced
- 2 cups sliced white mushrooms
- 2 cups peas, fresh or frozen and thawed
- 2 large carrots, chopped
- 3 garlic cloves, minced
- 1 teaspoon ground cumin

- ½ teaspoon garam masala
- ½ teaspoon sea salt
- ½ teaspoon freshly ground black pepper
- 1 tablespoon all-purpose flour
- 1 cup vegetable broth

Directions:

1. To make the potatoes: Bring a large pot of salted water to a boil. Add the potatoes and cook for 13 to 15 minutes, until tender. Drain.
2. In the bowl of a stand mixer fitted with the paddle attachment, or in a large bowl using an electric mixer, combine the cooked potatoes, butter, mayonnaise, salt, cumin seed, fennel seed, coriander, curry powder, garam masala, and cayenne. Mix on medium speed until creamy, being careful not to overmix. Taste and adjust the seasoning. Set aside.
3. To make the filling: In the skillet over medium heat, melt the butter. Add the onion and cook for 3 to 4 minutes, until it begins to soften. Stir in the mushrooms, spreading them evenly over the bottom of the skillet to prevent crowding. Cook for 4 to 5 minutes, stirring occasionally, or until the onion has browned. Stir in the peas, carrots, garlic, cumin, garam masala, salt, and pepper. Cook for 2 to 3 minutes, stirring once or twice.
4. Stir in the flour so it coats the vegetables, then stir in the broth. Cook for 5 to 7 minutes, or until the mixture comes to a steady simmer, then remove from the heat.
5. Preheat the oven to 400°F.
6. Spread the mashed potatoes in an even layer over the vegetables, making sure the potatoes kiss the side of the skillet.
7. Bake for 25 to 30 minutes, or until the potatoes are browned and bubbling.

106.Crunchy Parmesan And Garlic Zucchini

Servings: 4-6 Servings
Cooking Time: 20 Minutes

Ingredients:

- 3 tablespoons olive oil
- 4-6 small green zucchini, sliced into spears by cutting into ½ lengthwise and then into thirds
- Coarse salt and pepper
- 4 garlic cloves, sliced thin
- 1 cup panko crumbs, seasoned with salt, pepper and paprika
- 1 cup freshly grated parmesan or Romano cheese

Directions:

1. Preheat oven to 450 degrees.
2. Heat oil in a large cast iron skillet on medium-low heat.
3. Layer zucchini in skillet. Let brown on one side for 3 minutes and flip over pieces, browning as many spears as you can. Sprinkle with salt and pepper. Add sliced garlic and sauté for 1 minute.
4. Sprinkle panko crumbs and grated cheese on top. Transfer to oven until brown and bubbly, about 5-10 minutes.

Nutrition Info: Calories: 135, Sodium: 59 mg, Dietary Fiber: 2.4 g, Total Fat: 8.3 g, Total Carbs: 12.2 g, Protein: 3.6 g.

107.Sesame Cauliflower

Servings: 4
Cooking Time: 20 Minutes

Ingredients:

- FOR THE CAULIFLOWER
- ½ cup vegetable oil
- 1 egg
- ¼ cup cornstarch
- 1 tablespoon garlic powder
- 1 tablespoon sesame oil
- 1 tablespoon soy sauce
- 1 head cauliflower, cut into florets

- FOR THE SAUCE
- 1 tablespoon sesame oil
- 1" fresh ginger, peeled and finely chopped
- 3 garlic cloves, minced
- ¼ cup soy sauce
- ¼ cup honey
- 1 tablespoon rice vinegar
- 1 teaspoon sriracha
- ¼ cup water
- ½ tablespoon cornstarch
- TO SERVE
- 4 cups cooked rice
- 1 tablespoon sesame seeds
- Handful scallions, chopped

Directions:
1. Heat the oven to 200°F. Place a baking sheet inside it to warm.
2. In your skillet, heat the vegetable oil over medium-high heat to 375°F.
3. Whisk together the egg, cornstarch, garlic powder, sesame oil, and soy sauce. Dip the cauliflower florets in the batter one at a time, then drop them into the hot oil.
4. Fry for 3 to 4 minutes per side, until crispy and browned. Transfer to the baking sheet in the oven once they are done. Repeat with the remaining cauliflower.
5. In a medium bowl, whisk together all the ingredients for the sauce until fully combined, then set aside.
6. In a saucepan over medium heat, warm the sauce. When it is simmering, add the cauliflower to the sauce, stirring to coat. Cook for 3 to 4 minutes, until the sauce is thickened.
7. Plate a cup of rice and top with cauliflower. Sprinkle with sesame seeds and scallions to serve.

108.Penne With Tomatoes & White Beans

Servings: 4
Cooking Time: 30 Min
Ingredients:
- 8 ounces uncooked penne pasta
- 2 tablespoons olive oil
- 1 garlic clove, minced
- 2 cans (14 1/2 ounces each) Italian diced tomatoes, undrained
- 1 can (15 ounces) white kidney or cannellini beans, rinsed and drained
- 1 package (10 ounces) fresh spinach, trimmed
- 1/4 cup sliced ripe olives
- 1/2 teaspoon salt
- 1/4 teaspoon pepper
- 1/2 cup grated Parmesan cheese

Directions:
1. Cook the pasta according to package directions. Meanwhile, in a large skillet, heat oil over medium-high heat. Add garlic; cook and stir for 1 minute. Add tomatoes and beans. Bring to a boil. Reduce the heat; simmer, uncovered, 5-7 minutes to allow flavors to blend.
2. Add the spinach, olives, salt and pepper; cook and stir over medium heat until the spinach is wilted. Drain pasta; top with tomato mixture and cheese.

109.Roasted Brussel Sprouts

Servings: 2
Cooking Time: 20 Minutes
Ingredients:
- ½ pound Brussel sprouts, trimmed, tough outer parts removed
- 1 ½ cloves garlic, minced
- ½ tsp. cider vinegar
- 1 ½ tbsps. olive oil

- Salt and pepper to taste
- 2 tbsps. pine nuts, toasted

Directions:
1. Preheat the oven to 350F.
2. Heat oil in the skillet. Place Brussel sprouts in the skillet and cook until brown. Add garlic, vinegar, oil, salt, and pepper.
3. Place skillet in the oven and cook for 20 minutes. Shake the skillet several times to ensure sprouts are not burning.
4. Remove from the oven. Sprinkle with toasted nuts and serve.

110.Squash Fajitas With Goat Cheese

Servings: 4
Cooking Time: 30 Min
Ingredients:
- 2 pounds yellow summer squash, sliced
- 1 large sweet onion, chopped
- 2 tablespoons olive oil
- 4 garlic cloves, minced
- 1 teaspoon pepper
- 1/2 teaspoon salt
- 8 flour tortillas (8 inches)
- 1 log (4 ounces) fresh goat cheese, crumbled
- 2 tablespoons minced fresh parsley

Directions:
1. In a large skillet, saute squash and onion in the oil until tender. Add the garlic, pepper and salt; cook 1 minute longer.
2. Spoon onto tortillas. Top with cheese and sprinkle with parsley. Fold in sides.

111.Lentil Bolognese

Servings: 4
Cooking Time: 1 Hour
Ingredients:
- 1 cup dried lentils
- 2 tablespoons olive oil
- 1 white onion, diced
- 1 celery stalk, diced
- 1 large carrot, diced
- ¼ cup tomato paste
- ½ cup whole milk
- 1 cup white wine
- 4 cups water
- 1 (28-ounce) can diced tomatoes
- 1 tablespoon fresh rosemary leaves, minced
- 1 teaspoon dried oregano
- 1 teaspoon dried thyme
- 1 teaspoon dried basil
- 1 teaspoon sea salt
- Tagliatelle or fettuccine noodles, cooked, for serving
- Grated Parmesan cheese, for serving

Directions:
1. At least 2 hours before you plan to start cooking, soak the lentils in water.
2. Heat the oil in the skillet over medium heat. Add the onion, celery, and carrot. Cook for 4 to 5 minutes, stirring frequently, or until the vegetables start to brown and soften.
3. Stir in the tomato paste and cook for 2 to 3 minutes, stirring, or just long enough for the tomato paste to caramelize.

56

4. Whisk in the milk and cook for 15 to 20 minutes, stirring, until it has cooked down by half.
5. Drain the lentils, add them to the skillet, and stir in the wine. Cook for about 10 minutes, stirring frequently, or until the liquid has mostly cooked down.
6. Stir in the water, tomatoes with their juices, rosemary, oregano, thyme, basil, and salt. Bring the sauce to a light boil. Reduce the heat to low and cook, uncovered, for 25 to 30 minutes, stirring occasionally.
7. Place the cooked noodles in a large bowl. When the lentils are cooked to your taste, spoon the sauce over the noodles, top with Parmesan cheese, and serve.

112.Pancetta And Asparagus With Fried Egg

Servings: 2-4 Servings
Cooking Time: 10 Minutes
Ingredients:
- 1 tablespoon olive oil
- ¼ pound pancetta
- 3 small shallots, sliced thin
- ½ pound asparagus, tough ends broke off, sliced into 1 inch pieces
- Salt and pepper
- 2 eggs

Directions:
1. Heat olive oil in a cast iron skillet over medium heat. Fry the pancetta, stirring frequently. Transfer to a plate.
2. Add shallots and cook for 2 minutes. Add asparagus pieces and sauté for several minutes. Sprinkle with salt and pepper and continue to watch closely that asparagus is browned and cooked through. Add pancetta back to the pan and stir together. Transfer to a plate.
3. Add a little oil if necessary and fry an egg in pan. Top asparagus pancetta mixture with fried egg and season with salt and pepper.

Nutrition Info: Calories: 229, Sodium: 687 mg, Dietary Fiber: 1.2 g, Total Fat: 17.6 g, Total Carbs: 3.4 g, Protein: 14.6 g.

113.Salsa Bean Burgers

Servings: 4
Cooking Time: 10 Min
Ingredients:
- 1 can (15 ounces) black beans, rinsed and drained
- 3/4 cup panko (Japanese) bread crumbs
- 1 cup salsa, divided
- 1 large egg, lightly beaten
- 2 tablespoons minced fresh cilantro
- 1 garlic clove, minced
- 2 teaspoons canola oil
- 4 whole wheat hamburger buns, split
- Sliced avocado, optional

Directions:
1. In a large bowl, mash beans. Mix in bread crumbs, 1/2 cup of salsa, egg, cilantro and garlic. Shape bean mixture into four patties; refrigerate 30 minutes.
2. In a large skillet, heat oil over medium heat. Cook the burgers 3-5 minutes on each side or until a thermometer reads 160°. Serve on buns with remaining salsa and avocado if desired.

114.Black Bean Burger

Servings: 4
Cooking Time: 15 Minutes
Ingredients:
- FOR THE PATTIES

- 1 small white onion, chopped
- 4 garlic cloves, halved
- 2 (15-ounce) cans black beans, drained, divided
- 1 teaspoon ground cumin
- 1 tablespoon Worcestershire sauce
- Hot sauce
- ½ cup crumbled feta
- 1 teaspoon chipotle powder
- ½ teaspoon cayenne
- 1 egg
- 1 cup all-purpose flour
- ½ cup bread crumbs
- 1 tablespoon butter
- 2 tablespoons olive oil
- FOR THE BURGERS
- 4 slices provolone cheese
- 4 hamburger buns
- 1 tablespoon butter
- 2 tablespoons mayonnaise
- Lettuce
- Tomato, thickly sliced
- ¼ red onion, thinly sliced

Directions:
1. In a food processor, combine the onion, garlic, and half the black beans. Blend until smooth.
2. In a large bowl, mix the black bean mixture with the remaining black beans, cumin, Worcestershire, a few shakes of hot sauce, feta, chipotle powder, cayenne, egg, flour, and bread crumbs. Form the mixture into four patties.
3. In your skillet, heat the oil over medium-high heat.
4. When the oil is hot, put the patties in the skillet. Cook for 5 minutes, add the butter to the pan, and flip. Top each burger with a piece of cheese. Cook for an additional 5 minutes until cooked through and crisp. Transfer to a plate in the microwave to keep warm.
5. While the burgers are cooking, spread the butter on the hamburger buns. Place them butter-side down on the skillet and toast for 1 to 2 minutes.
6. Spread the mayonnaise on the buns and layer a burger patty, lettuce, tomato, and onion. Serve hot.

115.Crispy Asian Green Beans

Servings: 2
Cooking Time: 5 Minutes
Ingredients:
- ½ tsp. peanut oil
- ½ pound green beans, ends trimmed
- 1 clove garlic, minced
- Coarse sea salt to taste
- ¼ tsp. toasted sesame oil

Directions:
1. Heat a skillet on medium heat and add the peanut oil until it shimmers. Add the garlic and cook for 30 seconds. Add the green beans and salt to the pan and roast until golden brown, about 4 minutes.
2. Drizzle the toasted sesame oil in the last minute of cooking.
3. Serve.

116.Seared Mushroom Medley

Servings: 6-8 Servings
Cooking Time: 15 Minutes
Ingredients:
- 2 pounds assorted mushrooms, such as white button, cremini, baby Portobello, oyster and shitake

- 1 yellow onion sliced thin
- 2 tablespoons butter
- 1 tablespoon olive oil
- 2 garlic cloves, minced
- 2 green onions, sliced thin

Directions:
1. Preheat oven to 475 degrees. Place cast iron skillet on middle rack in oven to heat for about 15 minutes.
2. Clean mushrooms with damp towel. Slice the mushrooms into mid-sized pieces. Remove pan from oven and place mushrooms in hot pan. Allow mushrooms to sear in hot pan for 5-8 minutes. Remove skillet and turn over mushrooms so that flip side browns.
3. Once mushrooms are seared, add onion, butter and olive oil. Return to oven for 5-7 minutes. Toss in garlic and return pan to oven for another minute. Remove sizzling skillet and garnish with sliced scallions.

Nutrition Info: Calories: 73, Sodium: 28 mg, Dietary Fiber: 1.5 g, Total Fat: 5.0 g, Total Carbs: 5.5 g, Protein: 3.9 g.

117.Skillet Pasta Bake With Tomatoes And Cheese

Servings: 2
Cooking Time: 30 Minutes
Ingredients:
- 1 tbsp. extra-virgin olive oil
- 1 garlic clove, minced
- 14-ounce canned diced tomatoes with their juice
- 7-ounce canned tomato sauce
- ½ tsp. kosher salt
- Black pepper to taste
- ½ cup water, if needed
- 6 ounces rotini or penne pasta
- ½ cup ricotta cheese
- ¼ cup freshly grated Parmesan cheese, plus more for garnish
- 1 ½ tbsps. chopped fresh basil

Directions:
1. Preheat the oven to 400F.
2. Heat the olive oil in a skillet. Add the garlic and cook for 2 minutes.
3. Stir in the tomatoes and their juice and the tomato sauce. Season with salt and pepper.
4. Increase heat to high. Cook and stir for 5 minutes. Add water if needed.
5. Add the pasta to the sauce and mix well. Spread the pasta out evenly. Then top with ricotta cheese. Sprinkle parmesan on top.
6. Bake in the oven for 20 minutes, or until the cheese is bubbly and golden brown.
7. Garnish and serve.

118.Black Bean And Avocado Tostadas

Servings: 4
Cooking Time: 10 Minutes
Ingredients:
- 2 (15-ounce) cans black beans, drained but reserving ¼ cup liquid
- 1 teaspoon ground cumin
- ½ teaspoon paprika
- ¼ teaspoon red pepper flakes
- 1 teaspoon sea salt, divided
- 12 cherry tomatoes, halved
- ½ red onion, minced
- Juice of 2 limes
- ½ cup fresh cilantro, minced
- 2 garlic cloves, minced
- ½ cup vegetable oil, for frying
- 4 corn tortillas

- ½ cup cotija cheese
- 1 cup shredded romaine lettuce (or your favorite salad green)
- 2 avocados, peeled, pitted, and sliced

Directions:

1. In a saucepan over medium heat, combine the black beans, reserved liquid, cumin, paprika, red pepper flakes, and ½ teaspoon of salt. Cook, stirring frequently, until warmed through.
2. Reduce the heat to low, and simmer while stirring occasionally.
3. In a medium mixing bowl, combine the tomatoes, onion, lime juice, cilantro, garlic, and a pinch of salt. Stir well to combine and set aside.
4. In your skillet, heat the vegetable oil over medium-high heat to 375°F.
5. One at a time, fry the tortillas until they are crisp and golden brown, 45 to 60 seconds on each side. Transfer to a rack, sprinkle with salt, and allow to cool.
6. Use a fork to gently mash the black beans and remove them from the heat.
7. Plate each tortilla and top with a layer of black beans, cojita, lettuce, avocado, and salsa. Serve immediately.

119.Pinto Bean Tostadas

Servings: 6
Cooking Time: 30 Min
Ingredients:

- 1/4 cup sour cream
- 3/4 teaspoon grated lime peel
- 1/4 teaspoon ground cumin
- 1/2 teaspoon salt, divided
- 2 tablespoons canola oil, divided
- 2 garlic cloves, minced
- 2 cans (15 ounces each) pinto beans, rinsed and drained
- 1 to 2 teaspoons hot pepper sauce
- 1 teaspoon chili powder
- 6 corn tortillas (6 inches)
- 2 cups shredded lettuce
- 1/2 cup salsa
- 3/4 cup crumbled feta cheese or queso fresco
- Lime wedges

Directions:

1. In a small bowl, mix sour cream, lime peel, cumin and 1/4 teaspoon salt. In a large saucepan, heat 1 tablespoon oil over medium heat. Add garlic; cook and stir just until fragrant, about 45 seconds. Stir in beans, pepper sauce, chili powder and remaining salt; heat through, stirring occasionally. Keep warm.
2. Brush both sides of tortillas with remaining oil. Place a large skillet over medium-high heat. Add tortillas in two batches; cook 2-3 minutes on each side or until lightly browned and crisp.
3. To serve, arrange beans and lettuce over tostada shells; top with salsa, sour cream mixture and cheese. Serve tostadas with lime wedges.

120.Potato Au Gratin Bake

Servings: 6 Servings
Cooking Time: 1 Hour And 5 Minutes
Ingredients:

- 3 tablespoons unsalted butter
- 3 tablespoons flour
- ½ cup half and half
- ½ cup of milk
- 3 cloves minced garlic
- 1 teaspoon onion powder
- Salt and pepper to taste
- 6 medium Yukon Gold potatoes, peeled and thinly sliced, preferably using a mandolin
- 1 cup shredded Gruyere cheese

- 1 cup shredded Fontina cheese
- 1 bunch parsley, chopped finely

Directions:
1. Preheat oven to 450 degrees.
2. Heat a cast iron skillet over medium heat. Once hot, melt butter and add in the flour, whisking for 45 seconds. Add half and half, milk, garlic, onion powder, salt and pepper and whisk until smooth and not lumpy. Pour mixture into a separate bowl.
3. Place sliced potatoes in bottom of skillet in an overlapping pattern. Sprinkle both cheeses on top of each layer of potato. Pour milk mixture over potatoes, season with salt and pepper and sprinkle remainder of cheese on top. Cover with foil and bake for 45 minutes to 1 hour. Once potatoes are cooked, remove foil and bake in oven until top layer is golden brown. Remove from oven and sprinkle with parsley.

Nutrition Info: Calories: 355, Sodium: 278 mg, Dietary Fiber: 2.8 g, Total Fat: 18.0 g, Total Carbs: 36.2 g, Protein: 15.1 g.

121.Vegetarian Stir-fry

Servings: 2
Cooking Time: 15 Minutes
Ingredients:
- For the stir-fry sauce
- ⅓ cup soy sauce
- ¼ cup vegetable broth
- 1 tablespoon honey
- 2 teaspoons cornstarch
- For the stir-fry
- 2 tablespoons sesame oil
- 1 onion, diced
- 1 large carrot, cut into rounds
- 1 cup white button mushrooms, sliced
- 1 red bell pepper, cut into strips
- 1 yellow bell pepper, cut into strips
- 1 cup baby corn
- 1 cup sugar snap peas
- 1 cup fresh broccoli florets
- 3 garlic cloves, minced
- 1 teaspoon peeled, minced fresh ginger
- Cooked rice or noodles, for serving
- Minced scallion, for garnish

Directions:
1. To make the stir-fry sauce: In a small bowl, whisk the soy sauce, broth, honey, and cornstarch until the cornstarch dissolves.
2. To make the stir-fry: Heat the oil in the skillet over medium-high heat. Add the onion and cook for 1 to 2 minutes. Add the carrot and mushrooms and cook for 4 to 6 minutes. Add the red and yellow bell peppers, corn, snap peas, broccoli, garlic, and ginger. Cook for 2 to 3 minutes, stirring frequently.
3. Pour the sauce into the skillet and stir well to coat. Cook for 45 seconds to 1 minute, long enough for the sauce to thicken and coat the vegetables, then remove from the heat.
4. Serve over rice, garnished with scallion.

122.Mexican Grilled Cheese Sandwiches

Servings: 4
Cooking Time: 25 Min
Ingredients:
- 1 medium sweet yellow pepper, chopped
- 1 medium green pepper, chopped
- 2 teaspoons olive oil
- 8 slices rye bread

- 2 tablespoons mayonnaise
- 1 cup fresh salsa, well drained
- 3/4 cup shredded Mexican cheese blend
- 2 tablespoons butter, softened

Directions:
1.   In a small skillet, saute the peppers in oil until tender. Spread four bread slices with mayonnaise. Layer with peppers, salsa and cheese. Top with remaining bread. Butter outsides of sandwiches.
2.   In a small skillet over medium heat, toast the sandwiches for 2-4 minutes on each side or until cheese is melted.

123.Spring Pea And Mushroom Risotto

Servings: 4
Cooking Time: 1 Hour 10 Minutes
Ingredients:
- 4 tablespoons (½ stick) salted butter, divided
- 2 cups sliced button mushrooms
- 3 garlic cloves, minced
- 3 cups vegetable broth
- 1 tablespoon olive oil
- 1 white onion, minced
- Sea salt
- 1 cup Arborio rice
- ½ cup dry white wine
- Juice of 1 lemon
- ¼ cup grated Parmesan cheese
- 1 cup shelled peas, fresh or frozen, thawed to room temperature

Directions:
1.   In the skillet over medium heat, melt 1 tablespoon of butter. Add the mushrooms and cook for 4 to 5 minutes, stirring occasionally, or until the mushrooms are browned and tender. Stir in the garlic and cook for 1 minute. Transfer the mushrooms and garlic to a small bowl and set it aside.
2.   In a medium saucepan over high heat, bring the broth to a boil, then reduce the heat to low and let simmer for 20 minutes.
3.   In the skillet over medium heat, combine the oil and 1 tablespoon of butter. Add the onion and a pinch of salt and cook for 2 to 3 minutes, stirring occasionally, until the onion begins to soften.
4.   Add the rice to the skillet. Stir to thoroughly coat the rice with the oil and butter. Sauté for 1 to 2 minutes, stirring frequently to keep the rice from browning.
5.   Stir in the wine and cook, stirring, for 3 to 4 minutes, or until the wine is fully absorbed.
6.   Add 1 ladleful of warm broth to the rice, stirring constantly until the broth is absorbed. Repeat this process, adding broth one ladleful at a time and stirring while it fully absorbs, until all the broth has been added, which should take 25 to 30 minutes.
7.   Stir in the remaining 2 tablespoons of butter, the lemon juice, and Parmesan cheese.
8.   Add the cooked mushrooms and garlic and peas. Cook for 2 to 3 minutes. Taste and adjust the seasoning, if desired.

124.Miso-maple Roasted Brussel Sprouts

Servings: 4 Servings
Cooking Time: 25 Minutes
Ingredients:
- 2 tablespoons olive oil
- 1 pound Brussel sprouts, trimmed, tough outer parts removed, sliced in half
- 3 cloves garlic, minced
- ¼ cup white miso
- 1/8 cup apple cider vinegar
- ¼ cup maple syrup
- ¼- ½ cup water

Directions:
1. Heat cast iron skillet over medium heat. Place olive oil, garlic and Brussel sprouts in skillet. Cook undisturbed until nicely browned, 4-5 minutes.
2. Place in oven and continue cooking about 20 minutes until sprouts soften, shaking skillet occasionally.
3. Mix miso, vinegar, maple syrup and water together. Remove Brussel sprouts from oven and return to stovetop over low heat. Pour in miso mixture and stir until evenly coated. Cook on stovetop over low to medium heat until some of the liquid evaporates and thickens.
Nutrition Info: Calories: 200, Sodium: 672 mg, Dietary Fiber: 5.2 g, Total Fat: 8.5 g, Total Carbs: 28.9 g, Protein: 6.0 g.

125.Curried Acorn Squash And Rice Dinner

Servings: 2-4 Servings
Cooking Time: 1 Hour
Ingredients:
- 1 tablespoon olive oil
- 1 clove garlic, minced
- 1 small onion, diced
- 1 ½ cups acorn squash, peeled and cubed
- 1-2 tablespoons curry powder
- Salt and pepper
- ½ cup white rice
- 2 medium tomatoes, chopped
- ½ cup chickpeas, drained and rinsed
- ½ cup coconut milk
- 1 tablespoon tomato paste
- 1 cup vegetable broth

Directions:
1. Heat a cast iron skillet over medium heat. Add olive oil, garlic and onion and sauté several minutes. Add squash and sauté 5-6 minutes. Add curry powder, salt, pepper and rice into skillet and stir.
2. Add tomatoes, chickpeas, coconut milk and tomatoes paste to skillet and stir well. Cook until tomatoes start to break apart.
3. Pour in vegetable broth and bring to a boil. Reduce to low and continue to simmer until liquid reduces. Continue cooking until most of the liquid is absorbed by the rice and rice is tender, about 40-45 minutes. Serve in skillet.
Nutrition Info: Calories: 338, Sodium: 213 mg, Dietary Fiber: 8.4 g, Total Fat: 13.3 g, Total Carbs: 47.9 g, Protein: 10.1 g.

126.Ginger Kabocha Squash

Servings: 2
Cooking Time: 15 Minutes
Ingredients:
- 1 tbsp. oil
- ½ inch ginger, chopped
- Salt and pepper to taste
- 1 tsp. maple syrup
- ½ kabocha squash, peeled, seeded, and chopped

Directions:
1. Preheat the oven to 400F.
2. Heat oil in the skillet and add garlic. Cook for 2 minutes.
3. Toss squash in a bowl with salt, pepper, and maple syrup. Add squash to the skillet and cook for 2 minutes per side.
4. Cover skillet and place in the oven until squash cooks through, about 5 to 10 minutes.
5. Serve.

127.Linguine With Broccoli Rabe & Peppers

Servings: 6
Cooking Time: 25 Min
Ingredients:
- 1 pound broccoli rabe
- 1 package (16 ounces) linguine
- 3 tablespoons olive oil
- 2 anchovy fillets, finely chopped, optional
- 3 garlic cloves, minced
- 1/2 cup sliced roasted sweet red peppers
- 1/2 cup pitted Greek olives, halved
- 1/2 teaspoon crushed red pepper flakes
- 1/4 teaspoon pepper
- 1/8 teaspoon salt
- 1/2 cup grated Romano cheese

Directions:
1. Cut 1/2 in. off ends of broccoli rabe; trim woody stems. Cut stems and leaves into 2-in. pieces. Cook linguine according to package directions, adding broccoli rabe during the last 5 minutes of cooking. Drain, reserving 1/2 cup of the pasta water.
2. Meanwhile, in a large skillet, heat the oil over medium-high heat. Add anchovies and garlic; cook and stir 1 minute. Stir in red peppers, olives, pepper flakes, salt and pepper.
3. Add linguine and broccoli rabe to skillet; toss to combine, adding reserved pasta water as desired to moisten. Serve with cheese.

128.Fried Rice

Servings: 4
Cooking Time: 20 Minutes
Ingredients:
- 2 large eggs
- Pinch sea salt
- 3 tablespoons peanut oil, divided
- 1 white onion, chopped
- 1 large carrot, shredded
- 2 garlic cloves, minced
- 1 cup shiitake mushrooms, sliced
- ½ cup chopped snow peas
- 1 cup chopped broccoli
- 1 tablespoon grated fresh ginger
- ¼ teaspoon red pepper flakes
- 1 tablespoon toasted sesame oil
- 3 cups cooked white rice
- 2 tablespoons soy sauce
- ¼ cup coarsely chopped scallions

Directions:
1. In a small bowl, whisk the eggs together with a pinch of salt.
2. In your skillet, heat 1 teaspoon of oil over medium-high heat. Add the eggs, allowing them to coat the bottom of the skillet. Cook for 1 to 2 minutes, until they have begun to set. Use a spatula to free the eggs and flip. Cook for an additional 2 to 3 minutes until cooked through.
3. Transfer the eggs to a medium bowl. Cover and place in the microwave to keep warm.
4. Add 1 tablespoon of oil to the skillet and return it to the heat. Once the oil is hot, add the onion, carrot, and garlic to the skillet. Cook for 3 to 5 minutes, stirring occasionally, until the onions begin to brown.
5. While the onion mixture is cooking, coarsely chop the cooked eggs and return them to the bowl.
6. Add the mushrooms, snow peas, and broccoli to the pan. Cook for 3 to 5 minutes, until the vegetables begin to soften and brown. Remove the vegetables from the heat, mix them in with the eggs, and return the bowl to the microwave.

7.   Add the remaining oil to the pan and return to the heat. Add the ginger, red pepper flakes, sesame oil, and rice to the skillet. Cook for 3 to 4 minutes, stirring frequently, until the rice has warmed.
8.   Return the vegetables and egg to the skillet and add the soy sauce. Stir a few times to combine and then remove the pan from the heat. Mix in the scallions and taste to adjust the seasoning.
9.   Serve immediately.

129.Ricotta-stuffed Zucchini Boats

Servings: 4
Cooking Time: 20 Minutes
Ingredients:
- 1 cup ricotta
- ½ teaspoon sea salt
- Juice of 1 lemon
- 1 tablespoon fresh rosemary leaves
- 1 tablespoon fresh oregano leaves
- 2 large zucchini, halved lengthwise, seeds scooped out
- ½ cup shredded mozzarella cheese

Directions:
1.   Preheat the oven to 425°F.
2.   In a small bowl, stir together the ricotta, salt, lemon juice, rosemary, and oregano.
3.   Arrange the zucchini halves in the skillet, cut-side up. Evenly divide the filling among the 4 zucchini halves. Top each with about 2 tablespoons of mozzarella cheese.
4.   Bake for 15 to 20 minutes, or until the cheese is browned and bubbling. Let the zucchini boats cool slightly, then serve.

130.Buffalo-style Cauliflower

Servings: 2
Cooking Time: 25 Minutes
Ingredients:
- 1 tbsp. olive oil
- ½ head cauliflower, chopped into florets
- Salt and pepper to taste
- 1 tbsp. unsalted butter
- 2 tbsps. Frank's red-hot sauce
- ½ tbsp. fresh lime juice
- Chopped parsley or cilantro

Directions:
1.   Preheat the oven to 375F.
2.   Melt the butter in a bowl in the microwave. Add hot sauce and lime juice to the butter and mix.
3.   Heat a cast-iron skillet. Add oil and cauliflower florets. Cook for 5 minutes, or until browned. Pour in the hot sauce mixture and mix well.
4.   Place in the oven and cook for 15 to 20 minutes.
5.   Remove from the oven and garnish. Serve.

131.Spaghetti Pie

Servings: 6 Servings
Cooking Time: 30 Minutes
Ingredients:
- 1 pound sausage, any variety
- 3 garlic cloves, minced
- 28 ounce can crushed tomatoes
- ½ cup onion, finely diced
- ½ teaspoon sugar

- 1 teaspoon Italian seasoning
- 1 teaspoon salt
- ¼ teaspoon black pepper
- 2 cups water
- 8 ounces linguine
- 1 cup shredded mozzarella cheese
- 1 cup chopped basil

Directions:
1. Preheat oven to 400 degrees.
2. Heat cast iron skillet over medium heat. Add olive oil. Add sausage and garlic, breaking up sausage into pieces. Brown sausage and transfer to a plate.
3. Wipe out skillet and add tomatoes, onion, sugar, seasoning, salt and pepper. Sauté several minutes. Add water and spaghetti noodles and make sure sauce covers the noodles.
4. Bring to a boil and cook 9-12 minutes. Add in sausage and stir. Sprinkle cheese on top and bake in oven for 12-15 minutes or until cheese is bubbly.
5. Remove from oven and top with basil.

Nutrition Info: Calories: 482, Sodium: 1334 mg, Dietary Fiber: 4.5 g, Total Fat: 25.9 g, Total Carbs: 33.9 g, Protein: 27.8 g.

132.Gnocchi With Cherry Tomatoes And Basil

Servings: 6 Servings
Cooking Time: 15 Minutes
Ingredients:
- 1 pound store-bought gnocchi
- 2 tablespoons olive oil
- 2 cloves garlic, minced
- 1 pint yellow and red cherry tomatoes
- Coarse salt and pepper
- 1 cup fresh basil (loosely packed)
- ½ cup grated parmesan cheese

Directions:
1. Preheat oven to 400 degrees.
2. Heat a large pot of salted water and cook gnocchi according to package directions.
3. Heat a cast iron skillet over medium heat. Add olive oil and sauté garlic for 1 minute.
4. Add tomatoes, cooking until blistered, but not saucy. Sprinkle in a good amount of salt and pepper.
5. Stir in gnocchi and sprinkle basil and parmesan on top.
6. Transfer to oven and bake 8-10 minutes until bubbly.

Nutrition Info: Calories: 177, Sodium: 484 mg, Dietary Fiber: 2.2 g, Total Fat: 6.5 g, Total Carbs: 25.1 g, Protein: 4.5 g.

POULTRY RECIPES

133.Bacon & Rosemary Chicken

Servings: 4
Cooking Time: 30 Min
Ingredients:
- 4 boneless skinless chicken breast halves (5 ounces each)
- 1/2 teaspoon salt
- 1/4 teaspoon pepper
- 1/4 cup all-purpose flour
- 5 bacon strips, chopped
- 1 tablespoon butter
- 4 garlic cloves, thinly sliced
- 1 tablespoon minced fresh rosemary or 1 teaspoon dried rosemary, crushed
- 1/8 teaspoon crushed red pepper flakes
- 1 cup reduced-sodium chicken broth
- 2 tablespoons lemon juice

Directions:
1. Pound chicken breasts slightly with a meat mallet to uniform thickness; sprinkle with salt and pepper. Place flour in a shallow bowl. Dip chicken in flour to coat both sides; shake off excess.
2. In a large skillet, cook bacon over medium heat until crisp, stirring occasionally. Remove with a slotted spoon; drain on paper towels. Discard drippings, reserving 2 tablespoons in pan. Cook chicken in butter and reserved drippings 4-6 minutes on each side or until a thermometer reads 165°. Remove and keep warm.
3. Add garlic, rosemary and pepper flakes to skillet; cook and stir 1 minute. Add broth and lemon juice; bring to a boil. Cook until liquid is reduced by half. Return chicken and bacon to skillet; heat through.

134.Turkey Mole Tacos

Servings: 6
Cooking Time: 20 Min
Ingredients:
- 1 1/4 pounds lean ground turkey
- 1 celery rib, chopped
- 4 green onions, chopped
- 2 garlic cloves, minced
- 1 can (14 1/2 ounces) diced tomatoes, undrained
- 1 jar (7 ounces) roasted sweet red peppers, drained and chopped
- 2 ounces 53% cacao dark baking chocolate, chopped
- 4 teaspoons chili powder
- 1 teaspoon ground cumin
- 1/2 teaspoon salt
- 1/4 teaspoon ground cinnamon
- 1/4 cup lightly salted mixed nuts, coarsely chopped
- 12 corn tortillas (6 inches), warmed

Directions:
1. In a large nonstick skillet coated with cooking spray, cook the turkey, celery, green onions and garlic over medium heat until meat is no longer pink and vegetables are tender; drain.
2. Stir in the tomatoes, red peppers, chocolate, chili powder, cumin, salt and cinnamon. Bring to a boil. Reduce heat; cover and simmer for 10 minutes, stirring occasionally.
3. Remove from the heat; stir in nuts. Place about 1/3 cup filling on each tortilla.
4. FREEZE OPTION Freeze cooled meat mixture in freezer containers. To use, partially thaw in refrigerator overnight. Heat through in a saucepan, stirring occasionally and adding a little water if necessary.

135.Chicken Marsala

Servings: 4

Cooking Time: 35 Minutes
Ingredients:
- 1½ cups chicken broth
- 1½ cups Marsala wine
- 4 boneless, skinless chicken breasts, butterflied
- 2 tablespoons olive oil, plus more as needed
- ½ cup all-purpose flour
- 1½ teaspoons sea salt, divided
- 3 tablespoons salted butter
- 2 cups sliced cremini mushrooms
- 3 garlic cloves, minced
- ¼ teaspoon freshly ground black pepper
- 1 teaspoon fresh thyme leaves, minced
- 1 teaspoon fresh oregano leaves, minced
- ¼ cup heavy (whipping) cream
- Cooked angel hair pasta, for serving
- Minced fresh parsley leaves, for garnish
- Lemon wedges, for garnish

Directions:
1. In a medium saucepan over high heat, combine the broth and Marsala wine. Bring to a light boil, then reduce the heat to low and let simmer for 7 minutes.
2. On a cutting board and using a meat tenderizer, flatten the chicken to an even thickness.
3. Heat the oil in the skillet over medium-high heat.
4. In a shallow bowl, stir together the flour and ½ teaspoon of salt. Dredge both sides of the chicken in the flour. Place the chicken into the skillet and cook for 5 to 6 minutes, flip, and cook for 5 to 6 minutes more, adding more oil as needed. Set the chicken aside to cool.
5. In the skillet over medium heat, melt the butter. Add the mushrooms and cook for 5 to 6 minutes, stirring frequently, or until they are soft and begin to brown. Add the garlic and cook for 1 to 2 minutes, until fragrant.
6. Pour in the warm wine and broth mixture and stir in the pepper, thyme, oregano, and the remaining 1 teaspoon of salt. Cook for 2 to 3 minutes.
7. Stir in the cream and add the chicken to the skillet, flipping it once to coat. Simmer for 4 to 5 minutes, or until the sauce thickens.
8. Serve on a bed of angel hair pasta garnished with fresh parsley and a lemon wedge for squeezing.

136. Classic Italian Chicken

Servings: 4
Cooking Time: 45 Min
Ingredients:
- 1 large egg
- 1 tablespoon plus 1/4 cup water, divided
- 1/2 cup seasoned bread crumbs
- 1 broiler/fryer chicken (2 to 3 pounds), cut up
- 2 tablespoons canola oil
- 1 can (10 3/4 ounces) condensed tomato soup, undiluted
- 1/4 cup chopped onion
- 1/2 teaspoon garlic powder
- 1/2 teaspoon dried basil
- 1/2 teaspoon dried oregano
- 1 cup (4 ounces) shredded part-skim mozzarella cheese
- Shredded Parmesan cheese

Directions:
1. In a shallow bowl, beat egg and 1 tablespoon water. Place the bread crumbs in another shallow bowl. Dip chicken in egg mixture, then coat with crumbs. In a large skillet, cook chicken in oil over medium heat for 4-5 minutes or until browned; drain. Remove and keep warm.
2. In the same skillet, combine the soup, onion, garlic powder, basil, oregano and remaining water. Return chicken to pan. Cover and simmer for 40-45 minutes or until chicken juices run clear. Sprinkle with mozzarella cheese; cover and cook for 1-2 minutes or until cheese is melted. Sprinkle with Parmesan cheese.

137.Skillet Chicken Burritos

Servings: 8
Cooking Time: 30 Min
Ingredients:
- 1 cup (8 ounces) reduced-fat sour cream
- 1/4 cup chopped fresh cilantro
- 2 tablespoons chopped pickled jalapeno slices
- 2 teaspoons chopped onion
- 2 teaspoons Dijon mustard
- 1 teaspoon grated lime peel
- BURRITOS
- 2 cups cubed cooked chicken breast
- 1 can (15 ounces) black beans, rinsed and drained
- 1 can (11 ounces) Mexicorn, drained
- 1 cup (4 ounces) shredded reduced-fat cheddar cheese
- 1/4 teaspoon salt
- 8 whole wheat tortillas (8 inches), warmed
- Cooking spray
- Salsa, optional

Directions:
1. In a small bowl, combine the first six ingredients. In a large bowl, combine the chicken, beans, corn, cheese, salt and 1/2 cup sour cream mixture. Spoon 1/2 cup chicken mixture on each tortilla. Fold sides and ends over filling and roll up. Spritz both sides with cooking spray.
2. In a large nonstick skillet or griddle coated with cooking spray, cook the burritos in batches over medium heat for 3-4 minutes on each side or until golden brown. Serve with remaining sour cream mixture and salsa if desired.

138.Asparagus Turkey Stir-fry

Servings: 4
Cooking Time: 20 Min
Ingredients:
- 2 teaspoons cornstarch
- 1/4 cup chicken broth
- 1 tablespoon lemon juice
- 1 teaspoon soy sauce
- 1 pound turkey breast tenderloin, cut into 1/2-inch strips
- 1 garlic clove, minced
- 2 tablespoons canola oil, divided
- 1 pound fresh asparagus, trimmed and cut into 1 1/2-inch pieces
- 1 jar (2 ounces) sliced pimientos, drained

Directions:
1. In a small bowl, combine the cornstarch, broth, lemon juice and soy sauce until smooth; set aside. In a large skillet or wok, stir-fry the turkey and garlic in 1 tablespoon of the oil until meat is no longer pink; remove and keep warm.
2. Stir-fry asparagus in the remaining oil until crisp-tender. Add the pimientos. Stir broth mixture and add to the pan; cook and stir for 1 minute or until thickened. Return the turkey to the pan; heat through.

139.Thai Chicken Peanut Noodles

Servings: 6
Cooking Time: 30 Min
Ingredients:
- 1/4 cup creamy peanut butter

- 1/2 cup reduced-sodium chicken broth
- 1/4 cup lemon juice
- 1/4 cup reduced-sodium soy sauce
- 4 teaspoons Sriracha Asian hot chili sauce
- 1/4 teaspoon crushed red pepper flakes
- 12 ounces uncooked multigrain spaghetti
- 1 pound lean ground chicken
- 1 1/2 cups julienned carrots
- 1 medium sweet red pepper, chopped
- 1 garlic clove, minced
- 1/2 cup finely chopped unsalted peanuts
- 4 green onions, chopped

Directions:
1.   In a small bowl, whisk the first six ingredients until blended. Cook spaghetti according to package directions; drain.
2.   Meanwhile, in a large skillet, cook chicken, carrots, pepper and garlic over medium heat 5-6 minutes or until chicken is no longer pink, breaking up chicken into crumbles; drain.
3.   Stir in peanut butter mixture; bring to a boil. Reduce the heat; simmer, uncovered, 3-5 minutes or until the sauce is slightly thickened. Serve with spaghetti. Top with peanuts and green onions.

140.Chicken Portobello Stroganoff

Servings: 4
Cooking Time: 25 Min
Ingredients:
- 1 pound ground chicken
- 12 ounces baby portobello mushrooms, halved
- 1 medium onion, chopped
- 1 tablespoon olive oil
- 2 garlic cloves, minced
- 3 tablespoons white wine or chicken broth
- 2 cups chicken broth
- 1/2 cup heavy whipping cream
- 2 tablespoons lemon juice
- 1/4 teaspoon salt
- 1/8 teaspoon white pepper
- 1 cup (8 ounces) sour cream
- Hot cooked egg noodles or pasta

Directions:
1.   In a large skillet, cook the chicken, mushrooms and onion in oil over medium-high heat until meat is no longer pink. Add garlic; cook 1 minute longer.
2.   Stir in wine. Bring to a boil; cook until the liquid is almost evaporated. Add the broth, cream, lemon juice, salt and pepper. Bring to a boil; cook until liquid is reduced by half.
3.   Reduce heat. Gradually stir in sour cream; heat through (do not boil). Serve with noodles.

141.Turkey Fillets With Vegetables

Servings: 2
Cooking Time: 12 Minutes
Ingredients:
- 1 tbsp. olive oil
- 3 anchovy fillets
- 2 turkey fillets, 4–6 ounces each, pounded thin
- 1/8 cup chicken broth
- ½ tbsp. capers, chopped
- 1 tbsp. dill, chopped

Directions:
1. Heat oil in the skillet. Add the anchovies and cook for 5 minutes.
2. Place turkey fillets and cook for 3 minutes on each side. Remove cooked fillets to a plate.
3. Add the broth to the pan and deglaze the pan. Stir in the capers and cook for 1 minute.
4. Pour the sauce over the turkey fillets and sprinkle them with chopped dill. Serve.

142.French Onion Chicken

Servings: 2
Cooking Time: 45 Minutes
Ingredients:
- 1 tablespoon olive oil
- 2 boneless, skinless chicken breasts
- 1 tablespoon salted butter
- 2 large white onions, cut into slivers
- ½ cup dry white wine
- 1½ cups chicken broth
- 1 tablespoon cornstarch
- 4 garlic cloves, minced
- 1 tablespoon fresh thyme leaves
- 1 tablespoon fresh oregano leaves
- 1 teaspoon sea salt
- ½ teaspoon freshly ground black pepper
- 1 cup shredded Gruyère cheese, divided
- ½ cup grated Parmesan cheese
- Handful fresh parsley leaves, minced
- 1 lemon, cut into wedges

Directions:
1. Preheat the oven to 400°F.
2. Heat the oil in the skillet over medium heat. Add the chicken and cook for 5 minutes per side, or until browned. Remove the chicken from the skillet and set it aside.
3. Place the butter and onions into the skillet and cook for 5 to 6 minutes, stirring frequently, or until the onions are browned
4. Pour in the wine and cook for 1 to 2 minutes, stirring.
5. Whisk in the broth and cornstarch until smooth. Add the garlic, thyme, oregano, salt, and pepper.
6. Return the chicken to the skillet, turning it once to coat in the sauce. Top each chicken breast with ¼ cup of Gruyère cheese and ¼ cup of Parmesan cheese.
7. Bake for 15 to 20 minutes, or until the chicken's internal temperature reaches 165°F.
8. Using oven mitts, remove the skillet from the oven and set the broiler to high. Top each piece of chicken with ¼ cup of the remaining Gruyère. Broil for 2 to 3 minutes, or until browned and bubbling.
9. Top with fresh parsley and lemon juice and serve.

143.Gorgonzola & Orange Chicken Tenders

Servings: 4
Cooking Time: 25 Min
Ingredients:
- 1 large egg
- 1/4 teaspoon salt
- 3/4 cup seasoned bread crumbs
- 1 pound chicken tenderloins
- 2 tablespoons olive oil
- 1/4 cup orange marmalade, warmed
- 1/4 cup crumbled Gorgonzola cheese

Directions:
1. In a shallow bowl, whisk egg and salt. Place bread crumbs in another shallow bowl. Dip chicken in egg, then in bread crumbs, patting to help coating adhere to the tenderloins.

2.   In a large skillet, heat oil over medium heat. Add chicken; cook 3-4 minutes on each side or until chicken is no longer pink. Drizzle with warm marmalade; top with cheese. Remove from heat; let stand, covered, until cheese begins to melt.

144.Favorite Skillet Lasagna

Servings: 5
Cooking Time: 30 Min
Ingredients:
- 1/2 pound Italian turkey sausage links, casings removed
- 1 small onion, chopped
- 1 jar (14 ounces) spaghetti sauce
- 2 cups uncooked whole wheat egg noodles
- 1 cup water
- 1/2 cup chopped zucchini
- 1/2 cup fat-free ricotta cheese
- 2 tablespoons grated Parmesan cheese
- 1 tablespoon minced fresh parsley or 1 teaspoon dried parsley flakes
- 1/2 cup shredded part-skim mozzarella cheese

Directions:
1.   In a large nonstick skillet, cook sausage and onion over medium heat until no longer pink, breaking up sausage into crumbles; drain. Stir in spaghetti sauce, noodles, water and the zucchini. Bring mixture to a boil. Reduce heat; simmer, covered, 8-10 minutes or until noodles are tender, stirring occasionally.
2.   In a small bowl, combine ricotta cheese, Parmesan cheese and parsley. Drop by tablespoonfuls over pasta mixture. Sprinkle with the mozzarella cheese; cook, covered, 3-5 minutes longer or until cheese is melted.

145.Southwest Chicken Wrap

Servings: 2
Cooking Time: 30 Minutes
Ingredients:
- ½ tbsp. olive oil
- 1-pound chicken breasts, cut into strips
- ½ yellow onion, sliced
- 1 tsp. minced garlic
- ½ tsp. taco seasoning
- 7-ounce) canned black beans, drained and rinsed
- 7-ounce) canned corn
- 7-ounce jar salsa
- Salt and pepper to taste
- 2 (12-inch) flour tortillas
- Shredded lettuce
- ½ cup shredded Cheddar cheese or Mexican-style cheese blend
- Sour cream to taste

Directions:
1.   Heat oil in the skillet until hot.
2.   Add the chicken and cook for 5 minutes or until it starts to brown.
3.   Add the onion and cook until the chicken is cooked through, about 8 to 12 minutes more.
4.   Add the garlic, taco seasoning, black beans, corn, and salsa. Simmer until cooked through. Season with salt and pepper.
5.   Remove from the heat. Spoon over the tortillas and top each with lettuce, cheese, and sour cream. Serve.

146.Chicken Fajita Wrap

Servings: 2
Cooking Time: 25 Minutes

Ingredients:
- 1 tbsp. olive oil
- 2/3-pound chicken breasts, cut into strips
- 1/3 yellow onion, sliced
- 1/3 yellow bell pepper, cut into strips
- 1/3 green bell pepper, cut into strips
- 2 (12-inch) tortillas
- 1/3 tsp. garlic powder
- 1/6 tsp. onion powder
- 1/3 tsp. paprika
- 1/6 tsp. cayenne pepper
- 1/3 tsp. ground cumin
- Red pepper flakes to taste
- 1/3 tsp. sugar
- 2/3 cups Mexican-style cheese blend
- Salsa and sour cream to taste

Directions:
1. Heat the oil in the skillet.
2. Add the chicken and cook until it starts to brown. Add the onion and bell peppers and cook for 7 to 10 minutes, or until the veggies are done, and the chicken is cooked through.
3. Toast the tortillas directly on the grill grate for 2 to 3 minutes on each side.
4. Add the garlic powder, onion powder, paprika, cayenne, cumin, red pepper flakes, and sugar to the chicken and cook, for 3 to 5 minutes more or until well combined.
5. Remove from the heat. Divide the chicken mixture evenly among the tortillas and top with cheese, salsa, and sour cream. Serve.

147.Cilantro-lime Turkey Burgers

Servings: 2
Cooking Time: 15 Minutes
Ingredients:
- ½ pound ground turkey
- 2 tbsps. minced fresh cilantro leaves, plus more for serving
- ½ jalapeño pepper, minced
- 1 garlic clove, minced
- ½ tsp. minced peeled fresh ginger
- Pinch sea salt
- 2 tbsps. plus 1 tbsp. olive oil, divided
- 2 buns
- Juice of ½ lime
- 2 tbsps. shredded Gruyère cheese
- Handful dandelion greens

Directions:
1. In a bowl, mix the turkey, cilantro, jalapeno pepper, garlic, ginger, and sea salt.
2. Shape the turkey mixture into 2 patties.
3. Heat 2 tbsps. olive oil in a skillet.
4. Add the turkey patties and cook for 5 to 6 minutes per side. Remove the cooked burgers to a plate.
5. Preheat another skillet.
6. Brush the cut-side of the buns with the remaining 1 tbsp. oil and toast for 2 minutes.
7. Sprinkle the lime juice over the cooked burgers.
8. Assemble the burgers on the buns, topping each with the Gruyere, cilantro, and dandelion greens. Serve.

148.Turkey Stir-fry

Servings: 2
Cooking Time: 12 Minutes
Ingredients:
- ½ pound turkey meat, diced

- 1 tbsp. oyster sauce, divided
- ½-inch piece fresh ginger root, finely chopped, divided
- 1 tbsp Chinese cooking wine, divided
- ½ tbsp vegetable oil
- ½ tbsp minced garlic
- 6-ounce canned lychees, drained
- 1 red chile pepper, seeded and sliced into strips
- ½ tbsp soy sauce
- 1 dash ground black pepper, for garnish
- ½ bunch fresh cilantro, chopped, for garnish
- ½ bunch green onions, chopped, for garnish

Directions:
1. In a bowl, combine half of the Chinese cooking wine, half of the oyster sauce, and half of the ginger. Marinate the turkey in this mixture for 30 minutes.
2. Heat oil in a skillet and add garlic. Cook until browned.
3. Add the turkey with the marinade and the rest of the ingredients, except the garnishes.
4. Cook for 5 to 10 minutes or until cooked. Garnish and serve.

149.Miso Chicken Thighs

Servings: 2
Cooking Time: 45 Minutes
Ingredients:
- 2 tablespoons dark or red miso
- 2 tablespoons unsalted butter, at room temperature
- 1 tablespoon sesame oil
- 1 tablespoon peeled, minced fresh ginger
- 1 tablespoon minced garlic
- ½ teaspoon sea salt
- 4 boneless, skin-on chicken thighs

Directions:
1. Preheat the oven to 400°F.
2. In a small bowl, stir together the miso, butter, oil, ginger, garlic, and salt.
3. Rub the miso and butter paste evenly over the chicken thighs, working to get it under the skin whenever possible. Arrange the thighs in the skillet, skin-side down.
4. Roast for 40 to 45 minutes, or until the chicken skin is browned and the thickest part of the thigh reaches 165°F. Let it rest for 10 minutes before serving.

150.Speedy Chicken Marsala

Servings: 4
Cooking Time: 30 Min
Ingredients:
- 8 ounces uncooked whole wheat or multigrain angel hair pasta
- 4 boneless skinless chicken breast halves (5 ounces each)
- 1/4 cup all-purpose flour
- 1 teaspoon lemon-pepper seasoning
- 1/2 teaspoon salt
- 2 tablespoons olive oil, divided
- 4 cups sliced fresh mushrooms
- 1 garlic clove, minced
- 1 cup dry Marsala wine

Directions:
1. Cook pasta according to package directions. Pound chicken with a meat mallet to 1/4-in. thickness. In a large resealable plastic bag, mix the flour, lemon pepper and salt. Add chicken, one piece at a time; close bag and shake to coat.
2. In a large skillet, heat 1 tablespoon oil over medium heat. Add chicken; cook for 4-5 minutes on each side or until no longer pink. Remove from pan.

3. In the same skillet, heat the remaining oil over medium-high heat. Add mushrooms; cook and stir until tender. Add garlic; cook 1 minute longer. Add wine; bring to a boil. Cook for 5-6 minutes or until liquid is reduced by half, stirring to loosen browned bits from pan. Return chicken to pan, turning to coat with the sauce; heat through.
4. Drain the pasta; serve with chicken mixture.

151.Flavorful Chicken Fajitas

Servings: 6
Cooking Time: 5 Min
Ingredients:
- 4 tablespoons canola oil, divided
- 2 tablespoons lemon juice
- 1 1/2 teaspoons seasoned salt
- 1 1/2 teaspoons dried oregano
- 1 1/2 teaspoons ground cumin
- 1 teaspoon garlic powder
- 1/2 teaspoon chili powder
- 1/2 teaspoon paprika
- 1/2 teaspoon crushed red pepper flakes, optional
- 1 1/2 pounds boneless skinless chicken breast, cut into thin strips
- 1/2 medium sweet red pepper, julienned
- 1/2 medium green pepper, julienned
- 4 green onions, thinly sliced
- 1/2 cup chopped onion
- 6 flour tortillas (8 inches), warmed
- Shredded cheddar cheese, taco sauce, salsa, guacamole and sour cream

Directions:
1. In a large resealable plastic bag, combine 2 tablespoons oil, lemon juice and seasonings; add the chicken. Seal and turn to coat; refrigerate for 1-4 hours.
2. In a large skillet, saute peppers and onions in remaining oil until crisp-tender. Remove and keep warm.
3. Discard marinade. In the same skillet, cook chicken over medium-high heat for 5-6 minutes or until no longer pink. Return pepper mixture to pan; heat through.
4. Spoon filling down the center of tortillas; fold in half. Serve with cheese, taco sauce, salsa, guacamole and sour cream.

152.Turkey Penne With Lemon Cream Sauce

Servings: 4
Cooking Time: 30 Min
Ingredients:
- 2 cups uncooked penne pasta
- 1/2 pound turkey breast cutlets, cut into 3/4-inch pieces
- 3 tablespoons butter, divided
- 2 cups fresh broccoli florets
- 3 small carrots, thinly sliced
- 2 garlic cloves, minced
- 2 tablespoons all-purpose flour
- 1 1/2 teaspoons chicken bouillon granules
- 1/2 teaspoon dried thyme
- 1/4 teaspoon pepper
- 1/8 teaspoon salt
- 2 1/2 cups half-and-half cream
- 1/4 cup lemon juice
- 2 plum tomatoes, seeded and chopped

Directions:
1. Cook pasta according to package directions. Meanwhile, in a large skillet, saute turkey in 1 tablespoon butter until no longer pink. Remove from skillet and keep warm.

2.   In the same skillet, saute broccoli and carrots in remaining butter until crisp-tender. Add garlic; cook 1 minute longer. Stir in the flour, bouillon granules, thyme, pepper and salt until blended. Combine cream and lemon juice; gradually stir into broccoli mixture. Bring to a boil; cook and stir for 2-3 minutes or until thickened.
3.   Drain pasta; add to the skillet. Stir in turkey and tomatoes and heat through.

153.Bow Ties With Chicken & Shrimp

Servings: 7
Cooking Time: 15 Min
Ingredients:
- 5 1/4 cups uncooked bow tie pasta
- 3/4 pound boneless skinless chicken breasts, cubed
- 1 tablespoon butter
- 1 tablespoon olive oil
- 2 green onions, chopped
- 2 garlic cloves, minced
- 2 cans (14 1/2 ounces each) Italian diced tomatoes, undrained
- 2 tablespoons minced fresh parsley, divided
- 1 tablespoon each minced fresh basil, thyme and oregano or 1 teaspoon each dried basil, thyme and oregano
- 1/4 teaspoon pepper
- 2 teaspoons cornstarch
- 1/2 cup reduced-sodium chicken broth
- 3/4 pound cooked large shrimp, peeled and deveined
- 3 plum tomatoes, diced
- 10 large pitted ripe olives, sliced
- Minced fresh parsley

Directions:
1.   Cook pasta according to package directions. Meanwhile, in a large nonstick skillet, saute chicken in butter and oil until no longer pink. Add onions and garlic; cook 1 minute longer. Stir in the canned tomatoes, herbs and pepper.
2.   Combine cornstarch and broth until smooth; stir into the pan. Bring to a boil; cook and stir for 2 minutes or until thickened. Add the shrimp, plum tomatoes and olives; heat through. Drain pasta; serve with chicken mixture. Sprinkle with parsley.

154.Roasted Turkey Breast

Servings: 2 To 4
Cooking Time: 1 Hour 30 Minutes
Ingredients:
- 1 whole bone-in turkey breast
- 8 tablespoons (1 stick) butter, at room temperature
- 4 garlic cloves, minced
- 2 teaspoons sea salt
- 1 teaspoon chipotle powder
- 2 large onions, cut into rings
- ½ cup white wine
- ½ cup chicken broth
- Juice of 2 lemons

Directions:
1.   Clean the turkey breast and pat it dry. Let it come to room temperature, approximately 30 minutes. Do not let it sit out for more than 2 hours.
2.   Preheat the oven to 325°F.
3.   In a small bowl, stir together the butter, garlic, salt, and chipotle powder. Spread the butter mixture over the turkey, really working it into and under the skin wherever possible.
4.   Arrange the onions on the bottom of the skillet. Pour in the white wine and broth. Place the turkey on top of the onions.

5.   Roast for 1 hour 15 minutes to 1 hour 30 minutes, or until the skin is browned and crisp, the turkey's internal temperature reaches 165°F, and the juices run clear. Let it rest for 10 minutes before carving and serving.

155.Pan-roasted Turkey Wings

Servings: 2
Cooking Time: 1 Hour
Ingredients:
- 4 turkey wings, tips removed, and sections separated
- ½ tsp. salt
- 1 tbsp. oil
- 1 ½ cups ketchup
- 1 ½ cups apple juice
- 1 tsp. tabasco sauce
- ½ onion, chopped
- 4 garlic cloves, smashed
- 1 tsp. fresh thyme leaves

Directions:
1.   Preheat the oven to 300F. Place a rack in the middle of the oven.
2.   Sprinkle wing pieces with salt. Heat oil in a skillet. Add the wings and cook for 3 minutes on each side, or until lightly browned.
3.   Whisk the ketchup, apple juice, tabasco sauce, onion, garlic, and thyme in a bowl. Pour the sauce over the wings and place the pan in the middle of the oven.
4.   Cook for 30 minutes. Then flip and cook for 15 to 20 minutes more, or until the meat is tender and the sauce has thickened.
5.   Serve.

156.Turkey Curry

Servings: 4
Cooking Time: 20 Min
Ingredients:
- 1 cup sliced celery
- 1/2 cup sliced carrots
- 1 cup fat-free milk, divided
- 2 tablespoons cornstarch
- 3/4 cup reduced-sodium chicken broth
- 2 cups diced cooked turkey or chicken
- 2 tablespoons dried minced onion
- 1/2 teaspoon garlic powder
- 1 to 4 teaspoons curry powder
- Hot cooked rice, optional

Directions:
1.   Lightly coat a skillet with cooking spray; saute celery and carrots until tender. In a bowl, mix 1/4 cup milk and cornstarch until smooth. Add broth and remaining milk; mix until smooth.
2.   Pour over vegetables. Bring to a boil; cook and stir for 2 minutes or until thickened. Add the turkey, onion, garlic powder and curry powder; heat through, stirring occasionally. Serve with rice if desired.

157.Southwest Turkey Bulgur Dinner

Servings: 4
Cooking Time: 30 Min
Ingredients:
- 8 ounces lean ground turkey
- 1 small onion, chopped
- 1 garlic clove, minced

- 1 can (16 ounces) kidney beans, rinsed and drained
- 1 can (14 1/2 ounces) diced tomatoes with mild green chilies
- 1 1/2 cups water
- 1/2 cup frozen corn
- 1 tablespoon chili powder
- 1 teaspoon ground cumin
- 1/4 teaspoon pepper
- 1/8 teaspoon salt
- 1 cup bulgur
- TOPPING
- 1/2 cup fat-free plain Greek yogurt
- 1 tablespoon finely chopped green onion
- 1 tablespoon minced fresh cilantro

Directions:
1. In a large nonstick skillet coated with cooking spray, cook turkey and onion over medium heat until meat is no longer pink. Add garlic; cook 1 minute longer.
2. Stir in the beans, tomatoes, water, corn, chili powder, cumin, pepper and salt. Bring to a boil. Stir in bulgur. Reduce heat; cover and simmer for 13-18 minutes or until bulgur is tender.
3. Remove from the heat; let stand 5 minutes. Fluff with a fork. Meanwhile, in a small bowl, combine the yogurt, green onion and cilantro. Serve with turkey mixture.

158.Favorite Cola Chicken

Servings: 4
Cooking Time: 70 Min
Ingredients:
- 1 can (12 ounces) diet cola
- 1/2 cup ketchup
- 2 to 4 tablespoons finely chopped onion
- 1/4 teaspoon dried oregano
- 1/4 teaspoon garlic powder
- 8 bone-in chicken thighs, skin removed

Directions:
1. In a large skillet, combine first five ingredients. Bring to a boil; boil for 1 minute. Add chicken; stir to coat. Reduce the heat to medium; cover and simmer for 20 minutes.
2. Uncover skillet; simmer the mixture 45 minutes or until a thermometer reads 180°.

159.Chicken And Bacon Quesadilla

Servings: 2
Cooking Time: 20 Minutes
Ingredients:
- 2 (12-inch) tortillas
- ½ cup diced rotisserie chicken
- 2 slices bacon, cooked and diced
- ½ cups shredded Cheddar cheese or Mexican-style cheese blend
- 1 scallion, green and white parts, sliced
- 1 1/3 tbsps. ranch dressing
- 1 tbsp. olive oil

Directions:
1. On each tortilla, layer the chicken, bacon, cheese, and scallions. Drizzle with dressing and fold over, so the tortilla is flat.
2. Preheat the skillet over low heat for 2 minutes, then add the oil and heat for 2 minutes.
3. Toast each quesadilla for 3 to 5 minutes on each side, or until golden brown. Serve.

160.Thai Turkey Meatballs

Servings: 2
Cooking Time: 10 Minutes
Ingredients:
- 2 shiitake mushrooms
- ½ lb. lean ground turkey
- 1 tbsp. fish sauce
- ½ tbsp. ginger, grated
- 1/3 tbsp. green curry paste
- 1/3 tsp. sugar
- 1 egg, beaten
- 2 tbsp. green onions, finely chopped
- 2 tbsp. cilantro, finely chopped
- Salt and pepper to taste
- 1 tbsp. peanut oil

Directions:
1. Bring a pot of water to boil and pour over mushrooms in a bowl. Soak for 30 minutes and drain. Remove stems and chop the mushrooms.
2. In a bowl, mix mushrooms, turkey, fish sauce, ginger, curry paste, sugar, egg, green onions, salt, pepper, and cilantro and mix well.
3. Make meatballs from this mixture.
4. Heat peanut oil in a skillet and cook meatballs for 10 minutes or until golden brown.
5. Serve.

161.Jalapeno-bacon And Turkey Meatloaf

Servings: 2
Cooking Time: 35 Minutes
Ingredients:
- 8 oz. ground turkey
- 1 egg, beaten
- 3 tbsps. panko breadcrumbs
- 3 tbsps. red onion, chopped
- 1 jalapeño; seeded, ribbed and minced
- 2 tbsp. ketchup, plus 1 tbsp.
- ½ tbsp. Worcestershire sauce, plus a few dashes
- 1/2 tbsp. White vinegar
- 1 tsp. Dijon mustard
- ½ tsp. salt
- ½ tsp. pepper
- 1 tsp. honey
- 1 slice thick-cut bacon, halved

Directions:
1. Preheat the oven to 375F.
2. In a bowl, combine turkey, egg, breadcrumbs, onion, jalapeno, 1 tbsp. ketchup, 1/2 tbsp. Worcestershire sauce, vinegar, 1 tsp. mustard, salt, and pepper.
3. Form mixture into a ball and press into a greased cast-iron skillet.
4. In a bowl, combine remaining ketchup, Worcestershire sauce, mustard, and honey to make a glaze.
5. Spread half of the glaze on top of the meatloaf. Arrange bacon on meatloaf.
6. Place skillet in the oven for 25 minutes. Remove skillet and spread on remaining glaze and return to oven.
7. Bake for 5 minutes more.
8. Turn off the oven and turn the broiler on high. Place skillet under the broiler until bacon is crispy.
9. Cool, slice, and serve.

162.Chicken And Zucchini Curry

Servings: 4
Cooking Time: 40 Minutes

Ingredients:
- 1 tablespoon olive oil
- 1 pound boneless, skinless chicken breasts
- 1 tablespoon salted butter
- 1 large yellow onion, diced
- 4 garlic cloves, minced
- 1 tablespoon peeled, minced fresh ginger
- 1 tablespoon curry powder
- 1½ teaspoons paprika
- 1½ teaspoons ground cumin
- 1½ teaspoons garam masala
- ¾ teaspoon ground turmeric
- ¾ teaspoon ground coriander
- 1½ cups heavy (whipping) cream
- ½ cup chicken broth
- 1 (14.5-ounce) can crushed tomatoes
- 1 zucchini, chopped
- ½ teaspoon sea salt, plus more as needed
- 1 teaspoon cornstarch
- 2 cups cooked rice
- 1 avocado, peeled, halved, pitted, and sliced
- ¼ cup fresh cilantro
- 1 lemon, cut into wedges

Directions:
1. Heat the oil in the skillet over medium heat. Add the chicken and cook for 3 to 4 minutes. Flip the chicken and cook for 3 minutes more, or until both sides are browned. Transfer the chicken to a plate and set it aside.
2. Put the butter and onion into the skillet. Cook for 3 to 4 minutes. Add the garlic and cook for 1 minute, then add the ginger, curry powder, paprika, cumin, garam masala, turmeric, and coriander. Stir well to coat the onion.
3. Stir in the cream, broth, and crushed tomatoes. Bring the sauce to a light boil, then reduce the heat to low.
4. Roughly chop the chicken and add it to the skillet, along with the zucchini and salt. Let it simmer for 15 minutes, stirring occasionally. Taste and adjust the seasoning, if desired.
5. In a small bowl, stir together 2 tablespoons of sauce and the cornstarch until dissolved. Stir the slurry into the sauce, mixing well to fully incorporate. Cook for 10 minutes, stirring occasionally.
6. Serve over rice with avocado, cilantro, and a lemon wedge.

163.Turkey Burgers

Servings: 4
Cooking Time: 15 Minutes
Ingredients:
- 1 pound ground turkey
- 2 garlic cloves, minced
- 1 large egg, beaten
- 2 tablespoons Worcestershire sauce
- Pinch sea salt
- 2 tablespoons olive oil, plus more as needed
- 4 ounces fresh mozzarella cheese, sliced
- 2 tablespoons mayonnaise
- 4 hamburger buns
- Handful fresh spinach
- ½ red onion, thinly sliced

Directions:
1. In a medium bowl, mix the ground turkey, garlic, egg, Worcestershire sauce, and salt. Divide the mixture into 4 balls and shape them into patties.
2. Heat the oil in the skillet over medium heat.
3. Place the turkey patties into the skillet and cook for 5 to 6 minutes. Flip and top each burger with 1 slice of mozzarella cheese. Cook for 5 to 6 minutes more, until browned and the internal temperature reaches 165°F.

4.   Spread the mayonnaise on the cut side of the buns. Layer the turkey patty, fresh spinach, and onion on the bottom bun, cover with the top bun, and serve.

164.Cheesy Onion Chicken Skillet

Servings: 4
Cooking Time: 20 Min
Ingredients:
- 1 pound boneless skinless chicken breasts, cubed
- 2 teaspoons Mrs. Dash Garlic & Herb seasoning blend
- 2 tablespoons olive oil, divided
- 1 medium green pepper, cut into strips
- 1/2 medium onion, sliced
- 1 cup (4 ounces) shredded Colby-Monterey Jack cheese

Directions:
1.   Toss chicken with seasoning blend. In a large nonstick skillet, heat 1 tablespoon of the oil over medium-high heat. Add chicken; cook and stir 5-7 minutes or until no longer pink. Remove from pan. In same pan, add remaining oil, pepper and onion; cook and stir 3-4 minutes or until onions are crisp-tender.
2.   Stir in the chicken; sprinkle with cheese. Remove from the heat; let stand, covered, until the cheese is melted.

165.Turkey Sloppy Joes With Avocado Slaw

Servings: 6
Cooking Time: 20 Min
Ingredients:
- 1 pound ground turkey
- 1 medium onion, chopped
- 1 envelope sloppy joe mix
- 1 can (6 ounces) tomato paste
- 1 1/4 cups water
- SLAW
- 1 medium ripe avocado, peeled and cubed
- 1 tablespoon olive oil
- 2 teaspoons lemon juice
- 1/2 teaspoon ground cumin
- 1/4 teaspoon salt
- 1/4 teaspoon pepper
- 2 1/2 cups coleslaw mix
- 6 hamburger buns, split

Directions:
1.   In a large skillet, cook turkey and onion over medium heat 7-8 minutes or until the turkey is no longer pink and the onion is tender, breaking up turkey into crumbles; drain.
2.   Stir in sloppy joe mix, tomato paste and water. Bring to a boil. Reduce heat; simmer, uncovered, 8-10 minutes or until thickened, stirring occasionally.
3.   Meanwhile, place avocado, oil, lemon juice, cumin, salt and pepper in a blender; cover and process until smooth. Transfer to a small bowl; stir in coleslaw mix. Spoon meat mixture onto bun bottoms and top with slaw. Replace tops.

APPETIZERS AND SIDES

166.Sesame Broccoli

Servings: 2 To 4
Cooking Time: 10 Minutes
Ingredients:
- 4 tablespoons sesame oil, divided
- 1 head broccoli, separated into florets and halved
- 1 tablespoon soy sauce
- 3 garlic cloves, minced

Directions:
1. In your skillet, heat 2 tablespoons of sesame oil over medium-high heat.
2. Put the broccoli in the hot skillet, evenly distributing it across the bottom. Cook for 2 to 3 minutes without turning.
3. Flip the broccoli and add the soy sauce, remaining sesame oil, and garlic. Cover and cook for another 2 to 3 minutes.
4. Serve warm.

167.Spinach And Artichoke Dip

Servings: 4
Cooking Time: 40 Minutes
Ingredients:
- 1½ teaspoons olive oil
- 4 cups fresh spinach
- 3 garlic cloves, minced
- 2 cups artichoke hearts, frozen or canned and drained
- 8 ounces cream cheese, at room temperature
- ½ cup mayonnaise
- ¼ cup sour cream
- ½ cup grated Parmesan cheese
- ½ cup shredded white Cheddar cheese
- ¼ teaspoon sea salt
- ¼ teaspoon red pepper flakes
- Tortilla chips, for serving

Directions:
1. Preheat the oven to 375°F.
2. Heat the oil in the skillet over medium heat. Add the spinach and cook for 5 to 7 minutes, stirring frequently.
3. Add the garlic and cook for 2 to 3 minutes. Transfer the spinach to a large bowl.
4. Add the artichoke hearts, cream cheese, mayonnaise, sour cream, Parmesan cheese, Cheddar cheese, salt, and red pepper flakes to the spinach. Mix well. Spoon the dip into the skillet, spreading it evenly.
5. Bake for 25 to 30 minutes, or until the dip is bubbling and browned around the edges.

168.Skillet Greens

Servings: 2 To 4
Cooking Time: 40 Minutes
Ingredients:
- 1 bunch collard greens, cleaned and deveined (see tip)
- 1 tablespoon olive oil
- 1 small yellow onion, chopped
- 3 garlic cloves, minced
- ¼ cup apple cider vinegar
- 1 teaspoon sea salt

Directions:
1. Roughly chop the greens into bite-size pieces.

2.   Heat the oil in the skillet over medium heat. Add the onion and cook for 5 to 7 minutes, stirring occasionally, or until softened.
3.   Add the garlic and chopped greens to the skillet. Toss to coat, then add the vinegar and salt. Reduce the heat to medium-low and cook for about 30 minutes, stirring occasionally, until the greens are tender.
4.   Serve drizzled with the juice from the skillet.

169. Grilled Prosciutto-wrapped Radicchio With Dressing

Servings: 2
Cooking Time: 5 Minutes
Ingredients:
- ½ small heads radicchio, chopped
- 2 slices prosciutto, sliced in half lengthwise
- 1 tbsp. extra virgin olive oil
- 1 tbsp. balsamic vinegar
- Pepper to taste

Directions:
1.   Wrap each piece of radicchio tightly with a slice of prosciutto.
2.   Heat the oil in the skillet. Cook the radicchio for about 5 minutes.
3.   Remove from heat and drizzle with balsamic vinegar. Season with salt and pepper. Serve.

170. Savory String Beans

Servings: 2
Cooking Time: 25 Minutes
Ingredients:
- 4 bacon strips
- 2 cups cut green beans (1-1/2-inch pieces)
- 1 cup of water
- 1/2 cup chopped onion
- 2 tbsps. minced fresh basil
- 1 bay leaf
- 1/4 tsp. dill seed
- 1/4 tsp. garlic powder
- Salt to taste
- 1/8 tsp. pepper

Directions:
1.   Cook bacon until crisp in the skillet, about 5 minutes. Remove and crumble. Set aside. Drain, and reserve 1 tbsp. drippings.
2.   Add onion, seasonings, water, and beans to drippings. Bring to a boil and cook, uncovered for 15 to 20 minutes, or until beans are tender. Discard the bay leaf. Stir in the bacon and serve.

171. Grilled Swiss Cheese And Bacon Sandwich With Onions

Servings: 2
Cooking Time: 20 Minutes
Ingredients:
- 1½ tsps. oil
- 1 medium onion, sliced
- ½ cup beer of choice
- ¼ tsp. caraway seeds
- Salt and pepper to taste
- 4 slices firm white or multigrain bread, not thin sliced
- 2 tbsps. honey mustard or Dijon mustard
- 2 slices bacon, cooked
- 2 ounces thinly sliced Swiss cheese

- 1½ tbsps. unsalted butter, softened
- Cornichons, for garnish

Directions:
1. Heat oil in a skillet. Add the onion and cook for 5 minutes.
2. Add the beer and caraway seeds. Bring to a boil and cook until the beer is almost completely evaporated. Season with salt and pepper. Keep warm.
3. Heat another skillet on medium heat.
4. Meanwhile, lay the bread slices on a work surface in a single layer and spread each slice with mustard all the way to the edges. Place two slices of bacon on two of the slices and top with cheese. Cover the cheese with the remaining bread with the mustard side down, pressing slightly.
5. Spread half of the butter over the two sandwiches and lay them buttered-side down in the pan.
6. Lower heat and spread the remaining butter on the unbuttered tops. Cover with a lid that is slightly smaller than the pan.
7. Cook until the cheese is melted and bubbling, about 8 minutes. Turning the sandwiches halfway through.
8. Remove, cut in half, spoon the onions on top, garnish with cornichons and serve.

172.Vegetable Tempura

Servings: 4 To 6
Cooking Time: 15 Minutes
Ingredients:
- For the dipping sauce
- 1 cup dashi broth
- ¼ cup soy sauce
- 3 tablespoons mirin
- 1½ teaspoons sugar
- For the tempura
- Vegetable oil, for frying
- 1 cup all-purpose flour, divided
- Pinch sea salt
- 1 large egg, cold
- 1 cup cold water
- 1 sweet potato, cooked and thinly sliced
- 1 zucchini, thinly sliced into circles
- 1 cup oyster mushrooms, cut into strips
- 1 Japanese eggplant, thinly sliced into circles

Directions:
1. To make the dipping sauce: In a small saucepan over medium-high heat, combine the dashi, soy sauce, mirin, and sugar. Bring it to a boil, stir well, then remove it from the heat to cool.
2. To make the tempura: Heat 1 inch of oil to 350°F in the skillet over medium-high heat.
3. In a large bowl, combine the flour and salt. Carefully whisk in the egg, then the cold water, taking care not to overwhisk. A few lumps are fine.
4. Working in batches, dip the sweet potato, zucchini, mushrooms, and eggplant into the batter, coating completely, then place them into the skillet, making sure the vegetables aren't touching as you fry them. Fry for 2 to 3 minutes, flip, and fry for 1 minute more. Transfer the fried vegetables to a rack to cool slightly and repeat until all the vegetable are fried.
5. Serve warm with the dipping sauce.

173.Tuscan White Bean-cheese Dip With Pancetta

Servings: 2
Cooking Time: 10 Minutes
Ingredients:
- ¾ cup undrained canned cannellini
- 2 tbsps. broth
- 3 tbsps. small cubes pancetta
- ⅓ cup shredded creamy fontina (not aged)

- 1½ tbsps. grated Parmigiano-Reggiano
- ½ tbsp. Extra-virgin olive oil
- ½ tbsp. finely chopped sage leaves
- Salt and pepper to taste
- 4 thin slices of lightly toasted Italian bread rubbed with garlic and brushed with olive oil

Directions:
1. Puree the cannellini and broth in a food processor until smooth.
2. Heat a cast-iron skillet and add this mixture. Stir in the pancetta and cheeses until melted. Then add the olive oil and sage. Season with salt and pepper.
3. Serve with grilled bread slices.

174. Zucchini And Tomato Gratin

Servings: 4
Cooking Time: 20 To 25 Minutes
Ingredients:
- 2 large ripe tomatoes, cut into ¼" slices
- 1 large zucchini, cut into ¼" slices
- ¼ cup olive oil
- 3 garlic cloves, minced
- 1 cup grated Parmesan cheese
- ½ teaspoon sea salt
- 1 tablespoon fresh oregano, minced
- 1 tablespoon fresh thyme, minced

Directions:
1. Heat the oven to 375°F.
2. In your skillet, arrange the tomatoes and the zucchini in alternating rows, overlapping a little so they stand up.
3. Drizzle with the olive oil and top with the garlic.
4. In a small bowl, mix together the Parmesan, salt, oregano, and thyme. Sprinkle the mixture over the top of the vegetables.
5. Bake for 20 to 25 minutes, until the zucchini is cooked through and the cheese has formed a golden crust.
6. Serve warm.

175. Garlic Butter Green Beans

Servings: 2 To 4
Cooking Time: 10 Minutes
Ingredients:
- 3 tablespoons salted butter
- 1 pound fresh green beans, ends removed
- 2 garlic cloves, minced
- Pinch sea salt

Directions:
1. In the skillet over medium heat, melt the butter. Add the green beans and cook for 3 to 5 minutes, stirring occasionally.
2. Add the garlic and the salt, stir well, and cover the skillet. Cook for 5 minutes.
3. Serve with your favorite entrée.

176. Open-faced Egg Sandwiches

Servings: 2
Cooking Time: 5 Minutes
Ingredients:
- 4 egg whites
- 2 eggs

- 2 tbsps. grated Parmesan cheese
- 2 tsps. butter, softened
- 2 slices whole-wheat bread, toasted
- 1/8 tsp. dried rosemary, crushed
- 1/8 tsp. pepper

Directions:
1. Coat a skillet with cooking spray and heat over medium heat.
2. Whisk the egg whites, eggs, and cheese. Add to the skillet and cook until set.
3. Spread butter on one side of the toast. Add the egg mixture on top. Garnish with pepper and rosemary. Serve.

177.Thai-style Green Beans

Servings: 2
Cooking Time: 5 Minutes
Ingredients:
- 1 tbsp. reduced-sodium soy sauce
- 1 tbsp. hoisin sauce
- 1 tbsp. creamy peanut butter
- 1/8 tsp. crushed red pepper flakes
- 1 tbsp. chopped shallot
- 1 tsp. minced fresh gingerroot
- 1 tbsp. canola oil
- 1/2-pound fresh green beans, trimmed
- Chopped dry roasted peanuts and minced fresh cilantro (for garnish)

Directions:
1. In a bowl, combine the red pepper flakes, peanut butter, hoisin sauce, and soy sauce. Set aside.
2. In a skillet, cook ginger and shallot in oil for 2 minutes. Add green beans and cook for 3 minutes.
3. Add sauce mixture and mix. Sprinkle with peanuts and cilantro and serve.

178.Panzanella

Servings: 4
Cooking Time: 15 Minutes
Ingredients:
- ½ cup olive oil, divided
- 4 cups cubed baguette or sourdough bread
- 1 teaspoon sea salt, divided
- 3 garlic cloves, minced
- 2 shallots, thinly sliced
- 1 teaspoon Dijon mustard
- 2 tablespoons Champagne vinegar
- 2 pounds cherry tomatoes, halved
- 6 ounces fresh mozzarella cheese, cubed
- ½ cup fresh basil leaves, roughly chopped

Directions:
1. Heat ¼ cup of oil in the skillet over medium-low heat. Add the bread cubes and ½ teaspoon of salt. Cook for 10 to 12 minutes, tossing frequently, or until the bread is browned and crisp.
2. In a small bowl, whisk the remaining ¼ cup of oil, along with the garlic, shallots, mustard, and vinegar until frothy.
3. In a large bowl, combine the bread, tomatoes, and mozzarella. Toss with the vinaigrette and top with basil and the remaining ½ teaspoon of salt. Serve immediately.

179.Roasted Red Potatoes

Servings: 4 To 6

Cooking Time: 30 To 35 Minutes
Ingredients:
- 8 to 10 small to medium red potatoes, quartered
- ¼ cup olive oil
- 1 teaspoon sea salt
- 3 garlic cloves, minced
- 1 tablespoon coarsely chopped fresh rosemary
- 1 tablespoon coarsely chopped fresh oregano

Directions:
1. Heat the oven to 400°F.
2. In your skillet, combine the potatoes, olive oil, salt, garlic, rosemary, and oregano and toss to evenly coat.
3. Roast in the oven for 20 minutes, give the potatoes a good stir, and roast for another 10 to 15 minutes until cooked through and crisp.
4. Serve warm.

180.Fried Pickles

Servings: 4 To 6
Cooking Time: 15 Minutes
Ingredients:
- 1 cup all-purpose flour, plus 2 tablespoons
- 1 teaspoon paprika, divided
- 1 teaspoon sea salt, divided
- 1 teaspoon red pepper flakes, divided
- 2 large eggs
- ¼ cup apple cider vinegar
- 1 cup cornmeal
- Peanut oil or safflower oil, for frying
- 2 cups dill pickle slices, drained and patted dry

Directions:
1. On a work surface, line up 3 small bowls. In the first bowl, stir together 1 cup of flour, ½ teaspoon of paprika, ½ teaspoon of salt, and ¾ teaspoon of red pepper flakes.
2. In the second bowl, whisk the eggs and vinegar to combine.
3. In the third bowl, stir together the cornmeal and the remaining 2 tablespoons of flour, ½ teaspoon of paprika, ½ teaspoon of salt, and ¼ teaspoon of red pepper flakes.
4. Heat 1 inch of oil to 375°F in the skillet over high heat.
5. Dredge the pickle slices in the flour mixture, then in the egg mixture, and finally in the cornmeal mixture.
6. Working in batches, fry the pickles for 2 to 3 minutes per side, or until browned and crisp. Transfer them to a wire rack to cool slightly before serving.

181.Turmeric Roasted Beets

Servings: 4
Cooking Time: 40 Minutes
Ingredients:
- 4 large beets, peeled and chopped
- 2 tablespoons olive oil
- ¼ teaspoon ground turmeric
- Pinch sea salt

Directions:
1. Preheat the oven to 400°F.
2. In the skillet, combine the beets, oil, turmeric, and salt and toss well to coat.
3. Roast for 35 to 40 minutes, or until the beets are cooked through.
4. Serve warm or chilled.

182.Spicy Black Beans With Cotija

Servings: 2 To 4
Cooking Time: 15 Minutes
Ingredients:
- 1 tablespoon olive oil
- 1 yellow onion, minced
- 3 garlic cloves, minced
- 1 jalapeño pepper, seeded and minced
- 2 (15-ounce) cans black beans, drained
- ½ cup vegetable stock
- 1 teaspoon salt
- ½ teaspoon ground cumin
- ½ teaspoon chipotle powder
- ¼ teaspoon cayenne
- Juice of 1 lime
- ¼ cup cotija cheese, crumbled
- ¼ cup fresh cilantro, coarsely chopped

Directions:
1. In your skillet, heat the oil over medium heat.
2. Sauté the onion and garlic for 2 to 3 minutes, until softened. Add the jalapeño pepper and cook for another minute.
3. Add the black beans, vegetable stock, salt, cumin, chipotle, and cayenne. Stir well to combine and reduce the heat to low.
4. Simmer for 10 minutes, stirring frequently.
5. Remove from the heat and stir in the lime juice. Top with the cotija and cilantro to serve.

183.Parmesan And Parsley Smashed Potatoes

Servings: 2 To 4
Cooking Time: 1 Hour 15 Minutes
Ingredients:
- 7 to 10 small or medium red potatoes
- ¼ cup olive oil, divided
- 1 teaspoon sea salt, divided
- 1 teaspoon red pepper flakes, divided
- 4 tablespoons salted butter, cubed
- 2 garlic cloves, minced
- ½ cup grated Parmesan cheese
- ¼ cup curly parsley, minced

Directions:
1. Preheat the oven to 350°F.
2. In your skillet, toss the potatoes with 2 tablespoons of olive oil, ½ teaspoon of salt, and ½ teaspoon of red pepper flakes.
3. Transfer the skillet to the oven and roast the potatoes for 30 minutes, or until a fork easily penetrates the potatoes.
4. Remove the skillet and increase the oven temperature to 425°F.
5. Use a fork or meat tenderizer to smash the potatoes flat. Return the pan to the oven and roast for 25 minutes.
6. Remove the skillet from the oven. Flip the potatoes and top with the remaining olive oil, salt, red pepper flakes, and the butter, garlic, and Parmesan cheese.
7. Roast for 15 to 20 more minutes, until cooked through, brown, and crisp.
8. Top with the parsley and serve hot.

184.Backcountry Fry Bread

Servings: 2
Cooking Time: 20 Minutes

Ingredients:
- 2 cups all-purpose flour
- ¼ tsp. salt
- ½ tbsp. baking powder
- ½ tbsp. sugar
- ¾ cups warm water
- 1 ½ cups vegan shortening, divided, for frying

Directions:
1. In a bowl, mix the flour, salt, baking powder, and sugar to combine.
2. Add the warm water and mix. Then knead the dough a few times.
3. Preheat the skillet for 2 minutes. Move to low heat and add half of the shortening.
4. Shape the dough into 4 to 6 balls. Flatten each ball into a (½ inch) disk.
5. Fry the disks for 3 to 5 minutes per side. Transfer to a plate lined with paper towels. Repeat to finish.
6. Serve.

185.Roasted Cauliflower

Servings: 4
Cooking Time: 25 Minutes
Ingredients:
- 1 head cauliflower, cut into florets
- 2 tablespoons olive oil
- 1 teaspoon sea salt
- Juice of 1 lemon

Directions:
1. Preheat the oven to 450°F.
2. In the skillet, combine the cauliflower, oil, and salt and toss well to coat.
3. Roast for 20 to 25 minutes, or until the cauliflower is tender and browned.
4. Sprinkle it with lemon juice and serve.

186.Sweet Potato Fries With Blue Cheese

Servings: 2
Cooking Time: 15 Minutes
Ingredients:
- 1 tbsp. olive oil
- 1-1/4 pounds sweet potatoes, peeled and cut into 1/2-in.-thick strips
- 1 tbsp. apricot preserves
- 1/4 tsp. salt
- 3 tbsps. crumbled blue cheese

Directions:
1. Heat oil in a skillet. Cook the sweet potatoes for 15 minutes or until lightly browned. Add preserves and season with salt.
2. Top with cheese and serve.

187.Bacon Jalapeno Poppers

Servings: 4
Cooking Time: 20 Minutes
Ingredients:
- 4-ounce cream cheese, softened
- ½ cup finely shredded Cheddar cheese or Mexican-style cheese blend
- ½ tsp. seasoning salt
- ¼ tsp. black pepper
- ½ tbsp. vegetable oil
- 6 small jalapeños, tops cut off and seeds removed

- 6 slices bacon

Directions:
1. In a bowl, combine the cream cheese, cheddar cheese, seasoning salt, and pepper. Mix well.
2. Heat the oil in the skillet.
3. Spoon the filling into the jalapenos until each is ¾ full. Wrap 1 slice of bacon around each jalapeno and secure with toothpicks.
4. Place the jalapenos in the pan and cook for 5 to 8 minutes on each side or until the bacon is fully cooked.
5. Serve.

188.Sauteed Mushrooms With Hummus

Servings: 2
Cooking Time: 20 Minutes
Ingredients:
- 1/2 tbsp. olive oil, plus extra for drizzling
- 1/4 yellow onion, thinly sliced
- 4 ounces mushrooms, thinly sliced
- 1/2 tsp. minced garlic
- 1 cup hummus
- 1/4 tsp. ground cumin
- 1/4 tsp. paprika
- Salt and pepper to taste
- 1/4 lemon, for squeezing
- 1 tbsp. toasted pine nuts
- Parsley, chopped
- 2 pita pockets

Directions:
1. Heat the oil in the skillet.
2. Add the onion and cook for 8 t0 10 minutes or until translucent.
3. Add the mushrooms and garlic and cook for 5 to 10 minutes, or until mushrooms are cooked through.
4. Meanwhile spread, the hummus onto a plate.
5. Add the cumin and paprika to the mushroom mixture. Season with salt and pepper. Stir and remove from the heat.
6. Spoon the mushroom mixture over the hummus. Garnish with a drizzle of olive oil, lemon juice, pine nuts, and parsley. Sprinkle additional paprika and serve.

189.Collards And Black-eyed Peas

Servings: 4
Cooking Time: 40 Minutes
Ingredients:
- 1 cup black-eyed peas, soaked
- 2 tablespoons salted butter
- 1 white onion, diced
- 3 garlic cloves, minced
- 1 bunch collard greens, ribbed and thinly sliced
- ½ teaspoon salt
- 1 tablespoon apple cider vinegar
- ¼ teaspoon red pepper flakes

Directions:
1. Soak the peas for at least 4 hours before cooking—or overnight—in 2" of water. Drain and rinse.
2. In your skillet, melt the butter over medium heat.
3. Sauté the onion, stirring frequently, for 3 to 4 minutes. Add the garlic and collard greens to the pan. Stir occasionally to coat and cook for another 3 to 4 minutes.
4. Add the black-eyed peas, salt, vinegar, and red pepper flakes. Stir well and reduce the heat to low.
5. Cook for 20 to 25 minutes, stirring occasionally, until the beans have softened.
6. Season to taste before serving.

190.Hasselback Potatoes

Servings: 4 To 6
Cooking Time: 1 Hour
Ingredients:
- 5 Yukon gold potatoes
- 8 tablespoons (1 stick) salted butter, cubed
- 4 garlic cloves, minced
- 1½ teaspoons sea salt
- ½ teaspoon red pepper flakes
- Olive oil, for brushing
- ¼ cup grated Parmesan cheese
- 2 tablespoons fresh parsley leaves, minced

Directions:
1. Preheat the oven to 425°F.
2. Without cutting through the bottom skin, cut the potatoes crosswise into ½-inch slices. Arrange the potatoes in the skillet and sprinkle them with the butter, followed by the garlic, salt, and red pepper flakes.
3. Roast for 30 minutes.
4. Brush the potatoes with oil and bake for 30 minutes more.
5. Sprinkle the potatoes with Parmesan cheese and fresh parsley.

191.Roasted Root Vegetables

Servings: 4
Cooking Time: 40 To 45 Minutes
Ingredients:
- 1 large purple beet, peeled and cubed
- 1 large golden beet, peeled and cubed
- 1 sweet potato, peeled and cubed
- 5 small red potatoes, quartered
- 1 parsnip, peeled and cubed
- 5 carrots, peeled and sliced
- 1 yellow onion, diced
- ¼ cup olive oil
- 1 tablespoon herbes de Provence
- 3 garlic cloves, minced
- 1 teaspoon sea salt

Directions:
1. Heat the oven to 400°F.
2. In your skillet, combine the beets, potatoes, parsnip, carrots, and onion with the olive oil, herbes de Provence, garlic, and salt. Mix well to coat and spread the vegetables evenly over the skillet bottom.
3. Roast in the oven for 25 minutes, stir well, and roast for an additional 15 to 20 minutes. When the vegetables are cooked through and browning around the edges, remove from the heat.
4. Stir well to distribute the juices before serving.

192.Buffalo Wings

Servings: 4
Cooking Time: 40 Minutes
Ingredients:
- For the sauce
- 1 cup (2 sticks) salted butter
- 2 (5-ounce) bottles hot sauce
- 2 tablespoons Worcestershire sauce
- 1 tablespoon garlic powder

- For the wings
- 2 large eggs
- 2 tablespoons apple cider vinegar
- 1 cup all-purpose flour
- 1 cup bread crumbs
- 1 tablespoon garlic powder
- 1 tablespoon sea salt
- 1 tablespoon red pepper flakes
- Peanut oil, for frying
- 12 chicken wings and drumsticks, patted dry

Directions:
1.   To make the sauce: In a medium saucepan over medium-low heat, melt the butter. Whisk in the hot sauce, Worcestershire sauce, and garlic powder. Reduce the heat to low and simmer the sauce for 20 to 25 minutes, stirring occasionally.
2.   To make the wings: On a work surface, line up 2 small bowls. In the first bowl, whisk the eggs and vinegar.
3.   In the second bowl, stir together the flour, bread crumbs, garlic powder, salt, and red pepper flakes.
4.   Heat 1 inch of oil to 375°F in the skillet over high heat.
5.   Working one piece at a time, dip the chicken into the egg mixture, and then into the flour mixture. Working in batches of 3 or 4 at a time, carefully place the chicken in the hot oil and fry for 2 to 3 minutes per side, until cooked through and the juices run clear.
6.   Using tongs, remove the chicken from the skillet and dunk it in the hot sauce. Transfer the wings to a wire rack to cool slightly before serving.

193.Buttermilk Fried Okra

Servings: 4 To 6
Cooking Time: 15 Minutes
Ingredients:
- 2 cups all-purpose flour, divided
- 1 teaspoon sea salt, divided
- 1 teaspoon cayenne, divided
- 1 teaspoon garlic powder, divided
- 1 cup buttermilk
- 1 tablespoon apple cider vinegar
- 1 tablespoon hot sauce
- ½ cup bread crumbs
- Peanut oil, for frying
- 12 okra, cut into ½-inch slices

Directions:
1.   On a work surface, line up 3 small bowls. In the first bowl, stir together 1 cup of flour, ½ teaspoon of salt, ½ teaspoon of cayenne, and ½ teaspoon of garlic powder.
2.   In the second bowl, whisk the buttermilk, vinegar, and hot sauce to combine.
3.   In the third bowl, stir together the bread crumbs and the remaining 1 cup of flour, ½ teaspoon of salt, ½ teaspoon of cayenne, and ½ teaspoon of garlic powder.
4.   Heat 1 inch of oil to 375°F in the skillet over high heat.
5.   Dredge the okra slices in the seasoned flour, dip them in the buttermilk, and coat them in the seasoned bread crumbs.
6.   Working in batches, fry the okra for 2 to 3 minutes per side, or until browned and crisp. Transfer to a wire rack to cool slightly before serving.

194.Elote

Servings: 4
Cooking Time: 20 Minutes
Ingredients:
- 4 ears corn, shucked
- 2 tablespoons olive oil

- ½ cup mayonnaise
- ¾ cup crumbled cotija cheese, divided
- ½ teaspoon sea salt
- 1 teaspoon chipotle powder
- 1 garlic clove, minced
- ½ teaspoon cayenne
- ½ cup fresh cilantro, minced
- 1 lime, quartered

Directions:
1. Brush the corn with olive oil on all sides.
2. Heat your skillet over medium-high heat. Add the corn to the hot pan, turning every 3 to 4 minutes. Cook for 17 to 20 minutes, until all sides are slightly blackened and the corn kernels are bright yellow.
3. While the corn is cooking, mix the mayonnaise, ½ cup of cotija, salt, chipotle, and garlic. Spread it out in a thick layer on a large plate.
4. When the corn is done, roll each ear in the mayonnaise mixture. Top the corn with the remaining cotija, cayenne, and cilantro, being sure to turn to evenly coat each side.
5. Serve warm with a lime wedge.

195.Skillet Steak Sandwiches

Servings: 2
Cooking Time: 10 Minutes
Ingredients:
- 1 large onion, chopped
- 1 stick butter, divided
- 1 ½ garlic cloves, chopped
- 1 ½ pounds cubed steak
- Beef seasoning to taste
- ¼ cup Worcestershire sauce
- 2 sub rolls

Directions:
1. Melt half of the butter in a skillet. Add onion and cook for 3 to 5 minutes or until soft.
2. Add garlic and cook for 30 seconds. Remove the onion mixture from the pan and set aside.
3. Season the cubed steak with a beef seasoning.
4. Add the remaining butter and cook the beef until browned, about 5 to 6 minutes.
5. Add onion mixture, Worcestershire sauce, and mix.
6. Remove the beef mixture from the skillet.
7. Toast the rolls in the skillet.
8. Arrange the sandwiches and serve.

196.Charred Zucchini

Servings: 4
Cooking Time: 20 Minutes
Ingredients:
- 2 large zucchini, halved lengthwise
- 2 tablespoons olive oil
- ½ teaspoon sea salt, divided
- ¼ teaspoon freshly ground black pepper, divided

Directions:
1. Preheat the oven to 450°F.
2. Brush the zucchini on both sides with oil. Lay the zucchini, skin-side up, in the skillet and sprinkle with ¼ teaspoon of salt and ⅛ teaspoon of pepper.
3. Roast for 10 minutes, flip the zucchini, then roast for 5 to 7 minutes more, or until the zucchini are browned but still firm. Sprinkle with the remaining ¼ teaspoon of salt and ⅛ teaspoon of pepper and serve.

197. Balsamic Brussels Sprouts With Mozzarella And Pecans

Servings: 2 To 4
Cooking Time: 40 To 45 Minutes
Ingredients:
- 24 Brussels sprouts, trimmed and halved
- 1 tablespoon olive oil
- 1 teaspoon sea salt
- 1 tablespoon balsamic vinegar, plus a drizzle to finish
- 2 garlic cloves, minced
- 1 tablespoon butter
- ½ cup pecans, coarsely chopped
- 1 cup cubed fresh mozzarella

Directions:
1. Preheat the oven to 350°F.
2. In your skillet, toss the Brussels sprouts with the olive oil, salt, balsamic vinegar, and garlic.
3. Roast in the oven for 40 to 45 minutes, until the Brussels sprouts are tender.
4. While the sprouts are roasting, melt the butter in a small pan over medium-high heat. Add the pecans and, stirring frequently, cook for 2 to 3 minutes until toasted. Remove from the heat and set aside.
5. Transfer the Brussels sprouts to a bowl, and mix in the pecans and mozzarella. Drizzle with balsamic. Serve warm.

198. Butter Herbed Rice

Servings: 2
Cooking Time: 15 Minutes
Ingredients:
- 1 1/8 cups vegetable stock
- 1 cup instant white rice
- 1/2 tbsp. dried parsley
- 1/2 tsp. dehydrated chives
- 1/2 tsp. garlic salt
- 1/2 tbsp. unsalted butter
- Salt and pepper to taste

Directions:
1. Preheat the skillet for 2 minutes.
2. Put the vegetable stock, rice, parsley, chives, and garlic salt in the pan and mix.
3. Cook for 5 to 7 minutes, or until the mixture starts to boil.
4. Remove from the heat and add the butter, cover and let it sit for 5 minutes.
5. Remove the lid, stir and season with salt and pepper. Serve.

DESSERTS & SWEET

199.Plum Upside-down Cake

Servings: 8-10
Cooking Time: 40 Min
Ingredients:
- 1/3 cup butter
- 1/2 cup packed brown sugar
- 2 pounds fresh plums, pitted and halved
- 2 large eggs
- 2/3 cup sugar
- 1 cup all-purpose flour
- 1 teaspoon baking powder
- 1/4 teaspoon salt
- 1/3 cup hot water
- 1/2 teaspoon lemon extract
- Whipped cream, optional

Directions:
1. Melt the butter in a 10-in. cast-iron or ovenproof skillet. Sprinkle brown sugar over the butter. Arrange plum halves, cut side down, in a single layer over sugar; set aside.
2. In a large bowl, beat the eggs until thick and lemon-colored; gradually beat in sugar. Combine the flour, baking powder and salt; add to egg mixture and mix well. Blend water and lemon extract; beat into batter. Pour over plums.
3. Bake at 350° for 40-45 minutes or until a toothpick inserted near the center comes out clean. Immediately invert onto a serving plate. Serve warm with whipped cream if desired.

200.Iced Lemon Pound Cake

Servings: 6
Cooking Time: 1 Hour 15 Minutes
Ingredients:
- For the cake
- 2 cups (4 sticks) salted butter, plus 1 tablespoon
- 2½ cups granulated sugar
- 6 large eggs
- 1 teaspoon vanilla extract
- 3½ cups cake flour
- 2 teaspoons baking powder
- 1 teaspoon sea salt
- ¼ teaspoon ground mace
- 1 cup whole milk
- For the icing
- 1 cup powdered sugar
- Juice of 1 lemon

Directions:
1. To make the cake: Preheat the oven to 325°F. Grease the skillet with 1 tablespoon of butter.
2. In the bowl of a stand mixer fitted with the paddle attachment, or in a large bowl using an electric mixer, cream the butter until light and fluffy. Add the granulated sugar and continue beating. Mix in the eggs, one at a time, until fully incorporated. Mix in the vanilla.
3. In a large bowl, combine the flour, baking powder, salt, and mace. Add the dry ingredients to the wet ingredients, a little at a time, alternating with milk, until fully incorporated. Pour the batter into the skillet.
4. Bake for 1 hour 15 minutes, until browned on top and a toothpick inserted into the center comes out clean. Let the cake cool to room temperature.
5. To make the icing: In a small bowl, whisk the powdered sugar and lemon juice until smooth. Drizzle the icing over the pound cake before serving.

201.Walking Tacos

Servings: 5
Cooking Time: 30 Min
Ingredients:
- 1 pound ground beef
- 1 envelope reduced-sodium chili seasoning mix
- 1/4 teaspoon pepper
- 1 can (10 ounces) diced tomatoes and green chilies
- 1 can (15 ounces) Ranch Style beans (pinto beans in seasoned tomato sauce)
- 5 packages (1 ounce each) corn chips
- Toppings: shredded cheddar cheese, sour cream and sliced green onions

Directions:
1. In a large skillet, cook beef over medium heat 6-8 minutes or until no longer pink, breaking into crumbles; drain. Stir in chili seasoning mix, pepper, tomatoes and beans; bring to a boil. Reduce the heat; simmer, uncovered, for 20-25 minutes or until chili is thickened, stirring occasionally.
2. Just before serving, cut open corn chip bags. Add the beef mixture and toppings as desired.

202.Chocolate Pecan Pie

Servings: 6 To 8
Cooking Time: 30 Minutes
Ingredients:
- FOR THE CRUST
- 1¼ cups all-purpose flour
- ½ cup salted butter
- 1 tablespoon granulated sugar
- Pinch sea salt
- ¼ cup cold water
- FOR THE FILLING
- 3 eggs
- ½ cup brown sugar
- ½ cup granulated sugar
- ¼ teaspoon salt
- ¾ cup corn syrup
- 1 stick butter, melted
- 1½ cups chopped pecans
- 1 cup mini chocolate chips

Directions:
1. In a food processor or blender, combine the flour, butter, granulated sugar, and salt. Pulse until the mixture is crumbled and resembles coarse cornmeal.
2. While pulsing, add the water 1 tablespoon at a time until a ball forms. Wrap the dough in plastic wrap and chill for 1 hour.
3. Preheat the oven to 350°F.
4. In a large bowl, beat the eggs, then add the brown sugar, sugar, salt, corn syrup, and butter. Whisk together well. Stir in the pecans.
5. Roll out the dough on a floured work surface to a 15" round. Press into the bottom and sides of your skillet.
6. Sprinkle half the chocolate chips evenly over the bottom of the crust. Add half the filling (stirring just before pouring) to the skillet. Sprinkle on the remaining chocolate chips and top with the remaining filling.
7. Bake for 30 minutes. Let cool completely before serving.

203.Peach Cobbler

Servings: 8 Servings
Cooking Time: 1 Hour
Ingredients:
- 1 ½ cups all-purpose flour

- 1 teaspoon sugar
- ¼ teaspoon fine sea salt
- 1 stick cold butter, cut into pieces
- 5 to 6 tablespoons cold water
- ¼ cup all-purpose flour
- 1 cup light brown sugar
- ½ lemon, juiced
- 4 ½ cups peaches, sliced into thin wedges
- 3 tablespoons sugar
- 1 tablespoon cinnamon

Directions:
1. Preheat oven to 375 degrees.
2. To make the crust, mix flour, sugar and salt. Cut in butter with your fingertips. Add water, one tablespoon at a time until mixture is moist. Only pour enough water to make sure dough sticks together.
3. Place dough on a floured surface and roll out dough to one quarter inch thickness. Place dough in oiled 10 inch cast iron skillet. Pierce dough with fork. Bake for about 8-10 minutes or until browned. Remove from oven.
4. In a separate bowl, combine flour, brown sugar, lemon juice and peaches. Toss to coat thoroughly. Pour into prepared crust. Sprinkle with cinnamon-sugar mixture. Bake 40 minutes or until crust is golden and peaches are bubbly.

Nutrition Info: Calories: 328, Sodium: 146 mg, Dietary Fiber: 2.6 g, Total Fat: 12.0 g, Total Carbs: 53.5 g, Protein: 3.9 g.

204.Monster Skillet Cookie

Servings: 6 To 8
Cooking Time: 20 Minutes
Ingredients:
- 4 tablespoons butter, room temperature, plus more for greasing
- ¾ cup brown sugar
- ½ cup granulated sugar
- 2 eggs
- 1 cup peanut butter
- ½ teaspoon vanilla extract
- 1 teaspoon baking soda
- ¼ teaspoon sea salt
- 2 cups oats
- ½ cup candy-coated chocolates (I like M&M's brand)
- ¼ cup chocolate chips

Directions:
1. Preheat the oven to 350°F.
2. In the bowl of a stand mixer, or in a bowl with a hand mixer, cream together the butter, brown sugar, and sugar. Beat in the eggs, one at a time. Then beat in the peanut butter, vanilla, baking soda, and salt.
3. Add the oats to the mixture, then slow the mixer and add the M&Ms and chocolate chips.
4. Grease your skillet and scrape the batter into it. Gently spread the batter so it is even.
5. Bake for 15 to 18 minutes, until cooked through and crisp around the edges.
6. Allow to cool before serving.

205.Deep-dish Giant Double Chocolate Chip Cookie

Servings: 6-8 Servings
Cooking Time: 30 Minutes
Ingredients:
- ½ cup unsalted butter
- ½ cup light brown sugar
- ½ cup white sugar
- 1 teaspoon vanilla
- 1 large egg

- 1 cup all-purpose flour
- ½ teaspoon baking powder
- ½ teaspoon salt
- 1 cup chocolate chip
- ½ cup chocolate chunks

Directions:
1. Preheat oven to 350 degrees.
2. Preheat a 10 inch skillet. Melt butter over low heat.
3. Add sugars and stir well. Incorporate vanilla and egg, and beat quickly to make sure eggs do not cook. Stir in flour, baking soda and salt. Fold in chocolate chips and chunks and spread dough out in skillet lightly with a spatula to flatten.
4. Bake for 25 minutes until cookie appears browned on top.

Nutrition Info: Calories: 417, Sodium: 299 mg, Dietary Fiber: 1.4 g, Total Fat: 21.1 g, Total Carbs: 53.2 g, Protein: 4.9 g.

206. Strawberry, Lime, And Rhubarb Cobbler

Servings: 2
Cooking Time: 30 Minutes
Ingredients:
- 1 2/3 cups fresh ripe strawberries, cut in half
- 2/3 cup rhubarb, chopped finely
- 1/3 cup white flour
- 1/12 cup white milk
- 1 tbsp white sugar
- 1/12 cup butter, melted
- 1/3 egg, beaten
- ½ tsp baking soda
- 2/3 tbsp butter (for the skillet)

Directions:
1. Preheat the oven to 400F.
2. Melt 2/3 tbsp. butter in a skillet.
3. In a bowl, combine the strawberries, with sugar and add them to the skillet with the butter. Remove from the heat.
4. In a bowl, combine the flour, baking powder, and white sugar and whisk to mix. Add the melted butter, milk, and the beaten egg to the flour mixture and mix.
5. Spread the fruit into the bottom of the skillet and dollop the dough over the fruit mixture.
6. Bake at 25 minutes or until the dough has become golden brown and crunchy on top.
7. Rest for 10 minutes and serve.

207. Chocolate Cake With Whipped Hazelnut Icing

Servings: 6 To 8
Cooking Time: 35 Minutes
Ingredients:
- FOR THE CAKE
- 1 cup cocoa powder
- 2½ cups all-purpose flour
- 2 teaspoons baking powder
- 1 teaspoon baking soda
- 1 teaspoon salt
- ½ stick butter, room temperature
- 1½ cups granulated sugar
- 3 eggs
- ¼ cup vegetable oil
- 2 teaspoons vanilla extract
- 1 cup buttermilk

- 1 tablespoon butter, for greasing
- FOR THE ICING
- 1 stick butter, room temperature
- ¾ cup hazelnut spread
- 3 cups powdered sugar
- 1 teaspoon vanilla extract
- ¼ cup heavy cream

Directions:
1. Heat the oven to 350°F.
2. In a large bowl, sift together the cocoa, flour, baking powder, baking soda, and salt.
3. In the bowl of a stand mixer, or in a large bowl with a hand mixer, cream the butter and sugar.
4. In a small bowl, combine the eggs, oil, vanilla, and buttermilk.
5. Add ⅓ of the dry ingredients to the butter mixture while the mixer is running. When it is fully combined, add ⅓ of the wet ingredients and mix well. Continue, alternating wet and dry ingredients. Scrape the bottom of the bowl and mix for an additional 2 to 3 minutes.
6. Rub the butter on the bottom and sides of your skillet. Pour the batter into the skillet and bake for 30 to 35 minutes, until cooked through.
7. While the cake is baking, make the icing by combining the butter, hazelnut spread, sugar, and vanilla in the bowl of a stand mixer, or in a bowl with a hand mixer. Whip, slowly, adding the heavy cream to combine. Chill.
8. When the cake is done, let it cool to room temperature before icing. Spread the icing evenly over the top of the cake and serve.

208.Bourbon Pecan Pie

Servings: 8 Servings
Cooking Time: 2 Hours And 30 Minutes
Ingredients:
- ½ package refrigerated pie crust
- 1 tablespoon brown sugar
- 4 large eggs
- 1 ½ cups white sugar
- ½ cup melted butter
- ½ cup chopped toasted pecans
- 2 tablespoons all-purpose flour
- 1 tablespoon cream
- 1 ½ teaspoons bourbon
- ½ teaspoon vanilla extract
- 2 cups pecan halves

Directions:
1. Preheat oven to 350 degrees.
2. Form pie crust to fit a 10 inch greased cast iron skillet. Sprinkle with brown sugar. Pierce crust and bake for 10 minutes until golden brown.
3. Whisk eggs, white sugar, melted butter, chopped pecans, flour, cream, bourbon and vanilla extract in a large bowl. Pour into pie crust and top with pecan halves, arranged in concentric circles.
4. Transfer skillet to the oven and bake for 25-30 minutes. Turn oven off and let pie stand in oven with door closed for 2 hours.

Nutrition Info: Calories: 346, Sodium: 137 mg, Dietary Fiber: 0.6 g, Total Fat: 18.9 g, Total Carbs: 42.6 g, Protein: 4.1 g.

209.Red Velvet Crepe Cakes

Servings: 2 Crepe Cakes (8 Each)
Cooking Time: 25 Min
Ingredients:
- 1 package red velvet cake mix (regular size)
- 2 3/4 cups whole milk
- 1 cup all-purpose flour

- 3 large eggs
- 3 large egg yolks
- 1/4 cup butter, melted
- 3 teaspoons vanilla extract
- FROSTING
- 2 packages (8 ounces each) cream cheese, softened
- 1 1/4 cups butter, softened
- 1/2 teaspoon salt
- 12 cups confectioners' sugar
- 5 teaspoons vanilla extract
- Fresh blueberries

Directions:
1.   In a large bowl, combine the cake mix, milk, flour, eggs, egg yolks, butter and vanilla; beat on low speed for 30 seconds. Beat on medium for 2 minutes.
2.   Heat a lightly greased 8-in. nonstick skillet over medium heat; pour 1/4 cup batter into center of skillet. Lift and tilt pan to coat bottom evenly. Cook until the top appears dry; turn and cook 15-20 seconds longer. Remove to a wire rack. Repeat with remaining batter, greasing skillet as needed. When cool, stack crepes with waxed paper or paper towels in between.
3.   For frosting, in a large bowl, beat the cream cheese, butter and salt until fluffy. Add the confectioners' sugar and vanilla; beat until the frosting is smooth.
4.   To assemble two crepe cakes, place one crepe on each of two cake plates. Spread each with one rounded tablespoon frosting to within 1/2 in. of edges. Repeat layers until all the crepes are used. Spread the remaining frosting over tops and sides of crepe cakes. Garnish with blueberries.

210.Figgy Apple Brie Tart

Servings: 8
Cooking Time: 15 Min
Ingredients:
- 3 tablespoons butter, softened
- 3/4 cup sugar
- 2 large apples
- 1 cup dried figs, halved
- 1/2 pound Brie cheese, rind removed, sliced
- 1 sheet refrigerated pie pastry

Directions:
1.   Preheat oven to 425°. Spread butter over the bottom of a 10-in. cast-iron or ovenproof skillet; sprinkle evenly with sugar.
2.   Peel, quarter and core apples; arrange in a circular pattern over sugar, rounded side down. Place figs around apples. Place the skillet over medium heat; cook for 10-12 minutes or until sugar is caramelized and apples have softened slightly. Remove from heat; top with cheese.
3.   Unroll the pastry sheet; place over apples, tucking under edges. Place skillet in oven on an upper rack; bake 15-18 minutes or until crust is golden brown. Cool in pan 5 minutes. Carefully invert onto a serving plate; serve warm.

211.Cornmeal Towers With Strawberries & Cream

Servings: 12
Cooking Time: 5 Min/batch
Ingredients:
- 3 large egg whites
- 1 cup heavy whipping cream
- 1 cup cornmeal
- 1 cup all-purpose flour
- 1 1/2 teaspoons baking powder
- 1/2 teaspoon ground cardamom
- 1/4 teaspoon salt

- 1 1/4 cups 2% milk
- 1 cup whole-milk ricotta cheese
- 1/4 cup orange juice
- 2 tablespoons honey
- 1 teaspoon almond extract
- 1 to 2 tablespoons butter
- 1 pound fresh strawberries, sliced
- 2 tablespoons sugar

Directions:
1. Place the egg whites in a small bowl; let stand at room temperature 30 minutes. Meanwhile, in a small bowl, beat the cream until soft peaks form; refrigerate, covered, until serving.
2. In a large bowl, whisk the cornmeal, flour, baking powder, cardamom and salt. In another bowl, mix milk, ricotta cheese, orange juice, honey and extract until blended. Add ricotta cheese mixture to cornmeal mixture; stir just until moistened. With clean beaters, beat egg whites on high speed until stiff but not dry; fold into batter.
3. Heat a griddle or a large nonstick skillet over medium heat; grease with butter. Filling a 1/4-cup measure halfway with batter, pour batter onto griddle or skillet. Cook until edges begin to dry and bottoms are golden brown. Turn; cook until second side is golden brown. Cool the pancakes slightly.
4. In a bowl, toss strawberries with sugar. For each serving, stack three pancakes, layering each pancake with strawberries and whipped cream.

212.Fruity Dessert Crepe

Servings: 2
Cooking Time: 15 Min
Ingredients:
- 1/4 cup 2% milk
- 2 tablespoons beaten egg
- 3 tablespoons biscuit/baking mix
- 1 snack-size cup (3 1/2 ounces) vanilla pudding
- 1/2 small banana, sliced
- 2 tablespoons flaked coconut
- 1/4 teaspoon almond extract
- 3 fresh strawberries, sliced
- 1/2 medium kiwifruit, peeled and sliced

Directions:
1. In a small bowl, combine the milk and egg. Add biscuit mix and mix well. Heat a 10-in. nonstick skillet coated with cooking spray; pour batter into center of skillet. Lift and tilt pan to evenly coat bottom. Cook until top appears dry; turn and cook 15-20 seconds longer. Remove to a wire rack.
2. Transfer pudding to a small bowl; fold in the banana, coconut and extract. Spoon down center of crepe; fold sides over filling. Top with strawberries and kiwi.

213.Focaccia Barese

Servings: 8
Cooking Time: 30 Min
Ingredients:
- 1 1/8 teaspoons active dry yeast
- 3/4 cup warm water (110° to 115°), divided
- 1/2 teaspoon sugar
- 1/3 cup mashed potato flakes
- 1 1/2 teaspoons plus 2 tablespoons olive oil, divided
- 1/4 teaspoon salt
- 1 3/4 cups bread flour
- TOPPING
- 2 medium tomatoes, thinly sliced
- 1/4 cup pitted Greek olives, halved
- 1 1/2 teaspoons minced fresh or dried oregano

- 1/2 teaspoon coarse salt

Directions:
1. In a large bowl, dissolve yeast in 1/2 cup warm water. Add sugar; let stand for 5 minutes. Add the potato flakes, 1 1/2 teaspoons oil, salt, 1 cup flour and remaining water. Beat until smooth. Stir in enough of the remaining flour to form a soft dough.
2. Turn onto a floured surface; knead until smooth and elastic, about 6-8 minutes. Place in a greased bowl, turning once to grease the top. Cover and let rise in a warm place until doubled, about 1 hour. Punch dough down. Cover and let rest for 10 minutes.
3. Place 1 tablespoon olive oil in a 10-in. cast-iron or ovenproof skillet; tilt pan to evenly coat. Add dough; shape dough to fit pan. Cover and let dough rise until doubled, about 30 minutes.
4. With fingertips, make several dimples over top of dough. Brush with remaining tablespoon of oil. Blot the tomato slices with paper towels. Arrange the tomato slices and olives over dough; sprinkle with oregano and salt.
5. Bake at 375° for 30-35 minutes or until golden brown.

214.Ginger Mango Cobbler

Servings: 2
Cooking Time: 45 Minutes
Ingredients:
- 1 ½ cups mango, cubed
- ½ box of vanilla cake mix
- ¼ cup of water
- 1 tbsp honey
- ½ tbsp freshly grated ginger
- 1 egg
- ½ tsp vanilla extract
- ½ tbsp coconut oil
- ½ tsp allspice
- ½ tbsp butter

Directions:
1. Preheat the oven to 350F.
2. In a bowl, combine the cake mix with the egg and the water and set aside. Mix the mangoes, ginger, honey, butter, and allspice in another bowl.
3. Grease the skillet with coconut oil. Pour the mango mixture inside and add the cake mix, stirring gently to combine. Do not stir too much.
4. Bake in the oven for 35 to 40 minutes. Cool and serve.

215.Chocolate Chip Bread Pudding With Whiskey Sauce

Servings: 4 To 6
Cooking Time: 45 Minutes
Ingredients:
- FOR THE PUDDING
- ¼ cup salted butter, for greasing
- 1 loaf French bread, preferably a day old, broken into 1" pieces
- 1 cup chocolate chips
- 5 eggs
- 2 cups whole milk
- 1 cup heavy cream
- ½ cup sugar
- ¼ teaspoon ground cinnamon
- ¼ teaspoon ground nutmeg
- ¼ teaspoon ground ginger
- ¼ teaspoon vanilla extract
- FOR THE SAUCE
- 2 cups heavy cream
- 2 tablespoons salted butter

- ½ cup sugar
- ¾ cup whiskey
- 2 tablespoons cornstarch
- FOR THE CREAM
- 1 cup heavy whipping cream
- 1 tablespoon sugar
- 1 teaspoon vanilla extract

Directions:
1. Preheat the oven to 350°F.
2. Grease your skillet with the butter and evenly arrange the bread pieces inside. Sprinkle with the chocolate chips.
3. In a large bowl, whisk the eggs, milk, heavy cream, sugar, cinnamon, nutmeg, ginger, and vanilla. Pour over the top of the bread. Do not mix.
4. Bake for 45 minutes, remove from the oven, and cool, letting the filling set before serving.
5. While the pudding is in the oven, combine the cream, butter, and sugar in a saucepan over medium heat. Scald and reduce the heat to low.
6. Whisk together the whiskey and cornstarch and stir into the cream, stirring constantly until the sauce has thickened. Remove from the heat and set aside.
7. In a stand mixer, or with a hand mixer, combine the whipping cream, sugar, and vanilla. Whip on high until soft peaks form. Chill.
8. When the bread pudding comes out of the oven, drizzle with the whiskey sauce and serve with whipped cream on the side.

216.Grilled Fruit Medley

Servings: 4-6 Servings
Cooking Time: 5 Minutes
Ingredients:
- Cooking spray
- 2 tablespoons avocado oil
- 1 ½ tablespoon sugar
- ¼ teaspoon sea salt
- 2 large peaches or nectarines, cut into wedges
- 5 thick slices watermelon, with rind removed
- 3 thick slices pineapple, cut into sticks
- 2 teaspoons fresh lime juice
- 2 tablespoons chopped mint
- 1 cup blueberries

Directions:
1. Heat a cast iron skillet over medium high heat. Spray with cooking spray. Dab a small amount of oil onto fruit. Sprinkle on sugar and sea salt.
2. Place peach wedges, watermelon and pineapple into skillet, working in batches. Cook for 1-2 minutes on each side, until slightly charred and softened.
3. Place fruit on a platter and sprinkle with lime juice, chopped mint and blueberries.

Nutrition Info: Calories: 169, Sodium: 83 mg, Dietary Fiber: 3.8 g, Total Fat: 1.2 g, Total Carbs: 41.9 g, Protein: 2.7 g.

217.Crunchy Caramelized Bananas

Servings: 2
Cooking Time: 15 Minutes
Ingredients:
- 1 ½ tbsps. salted butter
- 2/5 cup loosely packed light brown sugar
- 1/8 cup water
- 1 ½ firm yellow bananas, peeled and sliced
- 1/8 cup dried cranberries

- 1/8 cup toasted pumpkin or sunflower seeds

Directions:
1. Preheat the skillet over low heat for 3 minutes.
2. Melt the butter in a bowl. Place the melted butter, brown sugar, and water in the pan and simmer for 3 to 5 minutes or until hot but not boiling.
3. Add the bananas and cook for 3 to 5 minutes or until the bananas soften.
4. Remove from the heat. Add the cranberries and seeds and gently stir until they are mixed in. Serve.

218.Sweet Cornbread Wedges

Servings: 8 Servings
Cooking Time: 20 Minutes
Ingredients:
- 1 stick unsalted butter
- 1 ½ cups ground yellow cornmeal
- ½ cup all-purpose flour
- 1 teaspoon baking powder
- ½ teaspoon baking soda
- 3 tablespoons granulated sugar
- ½ teaspoon salt
- 2 large eggs
- 1 ½ cups buttermilk
- ½ cup frozen corn, thawed

Directions:
1. Preheat oven to 400 degrees.
2. Melt 5 tablespoons butter in the microwave.
3. Whisk together cornmeal, flour, baking powder, baking soda, sugar and salt.
4. In a separate bowl, beat eggs until light and pale yellow. Whisk in buttermilk. Pour wet mixture into dry mixture and lightly incorporate until no dry streaks remain. Fold in melted butter until just combined. Add corn kernels.
5. Preheat cast iron skillet over low to medium heat. Place remaining 3 tablespoons butter in skillet and melt. Pour batter into the hot skillet and bake in oven until golden brown, about 15 minutes. Cut into wedges.
Nutrition Info: Calories: 204, Sodium: 375 mg, Dietary Fiber: 0.8 g, Total Fat: 13.4 g, Total Carbs: 17.7 g, Protein: 4.7 g.

219.Philly Cheesesteak Bites

Servings: 1 1/2 Dozen
Cooking Time: 5 Min
Ingredients:
- 1 package (22 ounces) frozen waffle-cut fries
- 1 medium onion, halved and sliced
- 1/2 small green pepper, halved and sliced
- 1/2 small sweet red pepper, halved and sliced
- 3 tablespoons canola oil, divided
- 1/2 teaspoon salt, divided
- 3/4 pound beef ribeye steak, cut into thin strips
- 1/4 teaspoon pepper
- 3 tablespoons ketchup
- 6 tablespoons process cheese sauce

Directions:
1. Bake 18 large waffle fries according to package directions (save remaining fries for another use). Meanwhile, in a large skillet, saute onion and peppers in 1 tablespoon oil until tender. Sprinkle with 1/8 teaspoon salt. Remove and keep warm.
2. In the same pan, saute steak in the remaining oil in batches for 45-60 seconds or until desired doneness. Sprinkle with pepper and remaining salt. On each waffle fry, layer the beef, onion mixture, ketchup and cheese sauce. Serve warm.

220.Buttermilk Pound Cake With Blackberry Jam

Servings: 6 To 8
Cooking Time: 1 Hour 15 Minutes
Ingredients:
- FOR THE CAKE
- 1 pound butter, plus more for greasing
- 1 teaspoon vanilla extract
- 2½ cups granulated sugar
- 6 eggs
- 3½ cups cake flour
- 2 teaspoons baking powder
- 1 teaspoon sea salt
- ¼ teaspoon mace
- 1 cup buttermilk
- FOR THE JAM
- 2 cups fresh blackberries
- 1 tablespoon sugar
- Juice of 1 lemon

Directions:
1.   Heat the oven to 325°F.
2.   In the bowl of a stand mixer, or in a bowl with a hand mixer, cream the butter until light and fluffy. Add the vanilla and sugar, and continue beating. Beat in the eggs, one at a time.
3.   In a large mixing bowl, sift the flour, baking powder, salt, and mace. Sift again.
4.   Add ⅓ of the dry ingredients to the wet ingredients and fully incorporate. Add ⅓ of the buttermilk and mix thoroughly. Repeat with the remaining ingredients, alternating dry ingredients and buttermilk.
5.   Grease your skillet with butter and pour in the batter, smoothing to evenly distribute.
6.   Bake for 1 hour and 15 minutes.
7.   While the cake is baking, combine the blackberries, sugar, and lemon juice in a small saucepan. Simmer, stirring occasionally, until the blackberries break down and a thick jam forms. Remove from the heat to cool.
8.   Allow the cake to rest for 15 minutes out of the oven before turning it out onto a plate. Top with the blackberry jam and serve warm.

221.Berry Buckle

Servings: 4 To 6
Cooking Time: 40 Minutes
Ingredients:
- ½ cup salted butter
- 1 cup all-purpose flour
- ½ cup sugar
- 1¼ teaspoons baking powder
- 1 teaspoon sea salt
- ¾ cup whole milk
- 1 teaspoon vanilla extract
- 1 cup fresh blueberries
- 1 cup fresh blackberries
- 1 cup fresh strawberries, hulled and quartered

Directions:
1.   Preheat the oven to 350°F.
2.   Add the butter to your skillet, and place it in the warming oven to melt.
3.   In a medium bowl, mix the flour, sugar, baking powder, salt, milk, and vanilla until combined.
4.   Remove the skillet from the oven and pour the batter over the melted butter. Do not mix!
5.   In a small bowl, combine the blueberries, blackberries, and strawberries. Pour on top of the batter. Do not mix!
6.   Bake for 40 minutes, until bubbling and cooked through.

222.Chili Con Queso El Dorado

Servings: 4 Cups
Cooking Time: 25 Min
Ingredients:
- 1 cup chopped green onions
- 1 tablespoon olive oil
- 1 garlic clove, minced
- 4 cans (4 ounces each) chopped green chilies
- 2 chipotle peppers in adobo sauce, finely chopped
- 2 cans (5 ounces each) evaporated milk
- 2 cups (8 ounces) shredded Monterey Jack cheese
- 1/4 cup minced fresh cilantro
- 1/8 teaspoon salt
- 2 to 4 drops hot pepper sauce
- Tortilla chips

Directions:
1.   In a large saucepan, saute the onions in oil until tender. Add garlic; cook 1 minute longer. Add the chilies and chipotle peppers; cook 2 minutes longer. Gradually stir in milk; heat through.
2.   Remove from the heat; stir in cheese until melted. Stir in the cilantro, salt and pepper sauce. Serve warm with tortilla chips.

223.Cran-apple Cobbler

Servings: 6-8
Cooking Time: 30 Min
Ingredients:
- 2 1/2 cups sliced peeled apples
- 2 1/2 cups sliced peeled firm pears
- 1 to 1 1/4 cups sugar
- 1 cup fresh or frozen cranberries, thawed
- 1/2 cup water
- 3 tablespoons quick-cooking tapioca
- 3 tablespoons Red Hots
- 1/2 teaspoon ground cinnamon
- 2 tablespoons butter
- TOPPING
- 3/4 cup all-purpose flour
- 2 tablespoons sugar
- 1 teaspoon baking powder
- 1/4 teaspoon salt
- 1/4 cup cold butter, cubed
- 3 tablespoons milk
- Vanilla ice cream

Directions:
1.   In a large, oven-safe skillet, combine the first eight ingredients; let stand for 5 minutes. Cook and stir over medium heat until mixture comes to a full rolling boil, about 18 minutes. Dot with butter.
2.   In a small bowl, combine the flour, sugar, baking powder and salt in a bowl. Cut in the butter until mixture resembles coarse crumbs. Stir in milk until a soft dough forms.
3.   Drop topping by heaping tablespoons onto hot fruit. Bake at 375° for 30-35 minutes or until golden brown. Serve warm with ice cream.

224.Flourless Mocha Cake

Servings: 2

Cooking Time: 45 Minutes

Ingredients:
- 1/8 cup caster sugar
- 1/6 cups dark chocolate
- 1/6 cup butter
- ½ shot of espresso
- 1 egg (yolk and whites separated)
- Icing sugar (for dusting)

Directions:
1. Preheat the oven to 360F.
2. Melt the chocolate and 2/3 of the butter in the microwave.
3. Once melted, add the egg yolks, half of the caster sugar, and Espresso shot until all sugar has dissolved.
4. In a bowl, mix the egg white until fluffy. Slowly incorporate the remaining sugar while beating. Pour the chocolate mixture into the egg whites and stir with a spatula to mix. Do not overbeat.
5. Grease the skillet with the remaining butter and pour the chocolate mixture into the skillet.
6. Bake for 40 to 45 minutes. Cool and serve.

225.Vinegar Pie

Servings: 6 To 8
Cooking Time: 45 Minutes

Ingredients:
- FOR THE CRUST
- 2½ cups all-purpose flour
- ¾ cup salted butter, cubed, plus more for greasing
- 3 tablespoons granulated sugar
- ¼ teaspoon sea salt
- ¼ cup cold water
- 1 egg, beaten
- FOR THE FILLING
- 1 cup sugar
- ½ cup brown sugar
- 2 tablespoons all-purpose flour
- 1 teaspoon ground ginger
- 1 teaspoon ground cinnamon
- 1 teaspoon ground nutmeg
- 1 teaspoon ground cardamom
- 5 eggs
- 1 stick butter, melted
- ¼ cup apple cider vinegar
- 1 teaspoon vanilla extract

Directions:
1. In a food processor or blender, combine the flour, butter, sugar, and salt. Pulse until the mixture is crumbled and resembles coarse cornmeal.
2. While pulsing, add the water 1 tablespoon at a time until a ball forms. Wrap the dough in plastic wrap and chill for 1 hour.
3. Preheat the oven to 325°F.
4. In a medium mixing bowl, combine the sugar, brown sugar, flour, ginger, cinnamon, nutmeg, and cardamom and mix well. Beat in the eggs, one at a time, then add the butter, vinegar, and vanilla.
5. Grease your skillet with butter.
6. Roll out the dough on a floured work surface to a 15" round. Press into the bottom and sides of the skillet.
7. Pour the filling into the crust. Bake for 45 minutes, until the pie is brown and mostly set. Allow to cool and set completely before serving.

226.Campfire Bundles

Servings: 6

Cooking Time: 15 Min
Ingredients:
- 1 large sweet onion, sliced
- 1 each large green, sweet red and yellow pepper
- 4 medium potatoes, cut into 1/4-inch slices
- 6 medium carrots, cut into 1/4-inch slices
- 1 small head cabbage, sliced
- 2 medium tomatoes, chopped
- 1 to 1 1/2 pounds smoked Polish sausage, cut into 1/2-inch slices
- 1/2 cup butter, cubed
- 1 teaspoon salt
- 1/2 teaspoon pepper

Directions:
1. Place the vegetables on three pieces of double-layered heavy-duty foil (about 18 in. square). Top with the sausage; dot with butter. Sprinkle with salt and pepper. Fold foil around mixture and seal tightly.
2. Grill, covered, over medium heat for 30 minutes. Turn and grill 30 minutes longer or until the vegetables are tender. Open foil carefully to allow the steam to escape.

227.Banana-pecan Clafouti

Servings: 8 Servings
Cooking Time: 45 Minutes
Ingredients:
- 1 cup whole milk
- ¼ cup whipping cream
- 3 eggs
- ½ cup granulated sugar
- 1 teaspoon vanilla extract
- 2 tablespoons butter, melted
- ¼ teaspoon salt
- ½ cup all-purpose flour
- 2 bananas, peeled and thinly sliced
- 2 teaspoons fresh lemon juice
- ½ cup pecans, roughly chopped

Directions:
1. Preheat the oven to 350 degrees.
2. Whisk together milk, cream, eggs, sugar, extract, butter and salt. Add the flour and whisk gently until incorporated.
3. Place sliced bananas in a bowl with lemon juice.
4. Lightly grease a cast iron skillet and heat in oven for 5 minutes. Remove skillet and pour in batter. Scatter bananas and pecans over batter and place in oven. Bake until golden and puffed, about 35 minutes.
Nutrition Info: Calories: 194, Sodium: 131 mg, Dietary Fiber: 1.1 g, Total Fat: 8.2 g, Total Carbs: 27.2 g, Protein: 4.5 g.

228.Zucchini Patties With Dill Dip

Servings: 2 Dozen (3/4 Cup Dip)
Cooking Time: 10 Min
Ingredients:
- 3/4 cup sour cream
- 2 tablespoons minced fresh dill
- 1 teaspoon lemon juice
- 1/8 teaspoon salt
- 1/8 teaspoon pepper
- 2 1/2 cups shredded zucchini
- 1 cup seasoned bread crumbs
- 1 teaspoon seafood seasoning

- 1/4 teaspoon garlic powder
- 1 large egg, lightly beaten
- 2 tablespoons butter, melted
- 1 large carrot, chopped
- 1/4 cup finely chopped onion
- 1/4 cup all-purpose flour
- 1/2 cup canola oil

Directions:
1. For dip, in a small bowl, combine the first five ingredients. Cover and refrigerate until serving.
2. Place zucchini in a colander to drain; squeeze to remove excess liquid. Pat dry; set aside.
3. In a large bowl, combine the bread crumbs, seafood seasoning and garlic powder. Stir in the egg and butter until blended. Add the carrot, onion and zucchini.
4. Place flour in a shallow bowl. Shape zucchini mixture into 24 small patties; coat with flour.
5. Heat oil in a large skillet; fry patties, a few at a time, for 3-4 minutes on each side or until lightly browned. Drain on paper towels. Serve with dip.

229.Chocolate Chip Cookie

Servings: 2
Cooking Time: 45 Minutes
Ingredients:
- 1 ½ cups all-purpose flour
- 1 ¼ cups semi-sweet chocolate chips
- ¾ tsp baking soda
- ¼ tsp salt
- 2/5 cup unsalted butter
- ¾ cup brown sugar
- ½ cup white sugar
- 1 ½ eggs
- 1 tbsp vanilla extract

Directions:
1. Preheat the oven to 350F. Grease a cast-iron skillet with butter.
2. Whisk the flour with salt and baking soda in a bowl.
3. Beat the eggs in another bowl with sugars until mixed. Add the vanilla extract and mix.
4. Add the dry flour mixture to the sugar mixture and stir well. Fold in the chocolate chips and stir to mix.
5. Press the cookie dough on the skillet and bake in the oven for 40 minutes.
6. Serve.

230.Individual Campfire Stew

Servings: 4
Cooking Time: 15 Min
Ingredients:
- 1 large egg, lightly beaten
- 3/4 cup dry bread crumbs
- 1/4 cup ketchup
- 1 tablespoon Worcestershire sauce
- 1 teaspoon seasoned salt
- 1 pound lean ground beef (90% lean)
- 2 cups frozen shredded hash brown potatoes, thawed
- 1 cup diced carrots
- 1 cup condensed cream of chicken soup, undiluted
- 1/4 cup milk

Directions:
1. Prepare grill for indirect heat. In a large bowl, combine the first five ingredients. Crumble beef over mixture and mix well. Shape into four patties. Place each patty on a greased double thickness of heavy-duty foil (about 12 in. square); sprinkle each with potatoes and carrots.

2.   Combine soup and milk; spoon over meat and vegetables. Fold foil around the mixture and seal tightly. Grill, covered, over indirect medium heat for 25-30 minutes or until meat is no longer pink and potatoes are tender. Open the foil carefully to allow steam to escape.

231.Vegan Carrot Cake

Servings: 2
Cooking Time: 25 Minutes
Ingredients:
- 1/4 lb. carrots, grated
- 1/8 coconut milk
- 1/8 cup of coconut sugar
- 1/8 cup unsweetened apple sauce
- 1/16 cup of coconut oil
- 1/8 tsp vanilla extract
- 1/2 cups wheat flour
- 1/2 tsp cinnamon
- 1/8 tsp ginger
- 1/2 tsp baking powder
- 1/4 tsp baking soda
- For the icing:
- ¼ can full-fat coconut milk
- ¼ tbsp maple syrup
- Cinnamon (for garnishing)

Directions:
1.   Keep the can of coconut milk in the fridge for 6 to 8 hours. Preheat the oven to 350F.
2.   Mix all the cake ingredients with the carrots and mix well.
3.   Pour the batter into a greased skillet and bake in the oven for 20 minutes.
4.   Meanwhile, prepare your icing by mixing everything with a hand mixer until soft and fluffy.
5.   Once the cake is baked, spread the icing on top and sprinkle with extra cinnamon on top. Serve.

OTHER FAVORITE RECIPES

232.Rosemary Buttermilk Biscuits

Servings: 6
Cooking Time: 25 Minutes
Ingredients:

- .
- 3 tablespoons salted butter, divided, plus 8 tablespoons (1 stick) cold salted butter, cubed
- 2 cups all-purpose flour, plus more for working the dough
- 1 teaspoon baking soda
- 2 teaspoons baking powder
- 1 tablespoon fresh rosemary leaves, finely chopped
- 1 teaspoon sea salt
- 1 cup buttermilk

Directions:
1.   Preheat the oven to 425°F. Grease the skillet with 1 tablespoon of butter.
2.   In a medium bowl, stir together the flour, baking soda, baking powder, rosemary, and salt.
3.   Using a fork or your clean hands, work the butter cubes into the flour mixture until the texture resembles coarse cornmeal. Stir in the buttermilk until a rough dough forms.
4.   Flour a work surface and place the dough on it. Pat the dough into a large rectangle. Fold the dough in half, turn it, and pat the dough into a large rectangle again. Repeat this process 3 or 4 times, folding and rotating the dough each time. Add flour as you work to keep the dough from sticking.
5.   Pat the dough 1½ to 2 inches thick. Use a 3-inch biscuit cutter or jar lid to cut the biscuits into rounds. Arrange the rounds in the skillet so they are nice and snug.
6.   Melt the remaining 2 tablespoons of butter and brush it over the top of the biscuits.
7.   Bake for 20 to 25 minutes, or until the biscuits are fluffy and golden brown.

233.Pita Bread

Servings: 8
Cooking Time: 25 Minutes
Ingredients:
- 1 cup warm water
- 2 teaspoons dry active yeast
- ½ teaspoon sugar
- 2 teaspoons sea salt
- 3 cups all-purpose flour, plus more for kneading
- 1 tablespoon olive oil, plus more for greasing

Directions:
1.   Coat a large bowl with olive oil and set aside.
2.   In a mixing bowl, combine the water, yeast, and sugar. Stir well and let the mixture sit for 10 minutes.
3.   Add the salt and slowly work in the flour, a little at a time, with a wooden spoon.
4.   When a rough dough ball has formed, turn it out onto a floured surface. Knead for 7 to 10 minutes, until the dough is smooth and elastic.
5.   Transfer the dough to the oiled bowl, turn once, and cover lightly with a towel. Allow the dough to rise in a warm place for 1 hour, until the dough has doubled in size.
6.   Gently punch down the dough and turn it out onto a floured work surface. Divide it into 8 equal pieces. Cover loosely with a towel and let it rest for 20 minutes.
7.   Gently form the pieces into discs, about 8" across and ¼" thick. Add extra flour to the dough as you work it to avoid sticking.
8.   Heat your skillet over medium-high heat. Add a little oil to the pan, and when the skillet is hot, cook your pitas one at a time. Cook for 1½ minutes per side, allowing the dough to puff up and brown.
9.   Transfer to a rack to cool and repeat with the remaining dough. Add oil to the skillet between each pita to avoid sticking.

234.Pull-apart Garlic Knots

Servings: 4 To 6
Cooking Time: 25 To 30 Minutes
Ingredients:
- FOR THE DOUGH
- 1½ tablespoons olive oil, plus more for greasing
- 1 tablespoon dry active yeast
- 1 tablespoon sea salt
- ¾ cup warm water
- 2½ cups bread flour, plus more for kneading
- FOR THE GLAZE
- 1 stick salted butter, melted
- 1 teaspoon sea salt
- 3 garlic cloves, minced
- FOR THE TOPPING
- ½ cup grated Parmesan cheese
- 1 tablespoon dried oregano

Directions:
1. Coat a large bowl with olive oil and set aside.
2. In another large bowl, whisk together 1½ tablespoons of olive oil, the yeast, salt, and water. Whisk until fully incorporated and frothing. Let sit for 10 minutes.
3. Add half the flour and stir the mixture with a wooden spoon. Add the remaining flour and use your hands to knead everything together. Knead for 10 minutes, until the dough ball is smooth and pliable.
4. Transfer the dough to the oiled bowl, turn once, and cover lightly with a towel. Allow the dough to rise in a warm place for 1 hour, until the dough has doubled in size.
5. Punch the dough down and allow it to rise for 15 more minutes.
6. Heat the oven to 400°F.
7. Gently turn the dough out onto a floured surface. Knead for 5 to 7 minutes, until the dough is pliable and stretches nicely without tearing.
8. Divide the dough into 16 even pieces. Roll each piece out into a 6" cylinder, adding flour as needed to keep the dough from sticking.
9. Tie each cylinder into a simple knot, tucking the ends under the bottom and arranging them in your skillet so they sit snugly next to each other.
10. In a small bowl, mix together the melted butter, salt, and garlic. Brush the knots generously with the garlic butter. Top with the Parmesan and oregano.
11. Bake for 25 to 30 minutes, until the knots rise and are golden brown.
12. Allow to cool slightly before serving.

235.Saucy Skillet Lasagna

Servings: 8
Cooking Time: 30 Min
Ingredients:
- 1 pound ground beef
- 1 can (14 1/2 ounces) diced tomatoes, undrained
- 2 large eggs, lightly beaten
- 1 1/2 cups ricotta cheese
- 4 cups marinara sauce
- 1 package (9 ounces) no-cook lasagna noodles
- 1 cup (4 ounces) shredded part-skim mozzarella cheese, optional

Directions:
1. In a large skillet, cook beef over medium heat 6-8 minutes or until no longer pink, breaking into crumbles; drain. Transfer to a large bowl; stir in tomatoes. In a small bowl, combine eggs and ricotta cheese.
2. Return 1 cup of the meat mixture to the skillet; spread evenly. Layer with 1 cup ricotta mixture, 1 1/2 cups marinara sauce and half of the noodles, breaking the noodles to fit as necessary. Repeat the layers. Top with the remaining marinara sauce.
3. Bring to a boil. Reduce heat; simmer, covered, 15-17 minutes or until the noodles are tender. Remove from heat. If desired, sprinkle with mozzarella cheese. Let stand for 2 minutes or until cheese is melted.

236.Cheddar-chive Biscuits

Servings: 2
Cooking Time: 20 Minutes
Ingredients:
- ½ cup all-purpose flour, plus more for kneading
- ¼ tsp. baking soda
- ¼ tsp. baking powder
- ¼ tsp. sea salt
- ¼ cup shredded cheddar cheese
- 1/8 cup minced fresh chives
- 2 tbsps. cold, salted butter, plus more for greasing
- ¼ cup buttermilk

Directions:
1. Preheat the oven to 425F.
2. In a bowl, mix the flour, baking soda, baking powder, salt, cheddar cheese, and chives.
3. Cut the butter into cubes and add it to the flour mixture. Mix with your hands, crumbling until the texture resembles coarse cornmeal.
4. Stir in the buttermilk.
5. Pat the dough on a floured work surface into a large rectangle. Fold the dough in half and turn and pat it out again into a large triangle. Repeat for 3 to 4 minutes.
6. Pat the dough out to 1 ½ to 2" thickness. Use a biscuit cutter to cut the biscuits into rounds.
7. Grease the skillet with butter. Arrange the dough rounds in the skillet toward the center so they are nice and snug.
8. Bake for 15 to 20 minutes or until golden.
9. Cool and serve.

237.Lemon Skillet Chicken

Servings: 4
Cooking Time: 10 Minutes
Ingredients:
- 1 cup all-purpose flour
- 3 lemons, 1 thinly sliced and 2 juiced, reserving 1 tablespoon zest
- 1 teaspoon sea salt, plus a pinch
- 2 boneless, skin-on chicken breasts, cut evenly in half
- 1 tablespoon olive oil
- 1 tablespoon butter
- 2 garlic cloves, minced

Directions:
1. In a small bowl, combine the flour, lemon zest, and 1 teaspoon salt. Dredge the chicken.
2. In your skillet, combine the olive oil, butter, and garlic over medium heat. Sauté for 2 to 3 minutes, until the garlic has browned.
3. Add the chicken to the skillet, searing for 3 to 4 minutes per side. Remove the skillet from the heat.
4. Top the chicken with the lemon slices and drizzle the lemon juice over the chicken. Sprinkle with salt and serve.

238.Blackened Grouper

Servings: 4
Cooking Time: 10 Minutes
Ingredients:
- 1 teaspoon dried oregano
- 1 teaspoon freshly ground black pepper
- 1 teaspoon sea salt

- ½ teaspoon cayenne
- ¼ teaspoon red pepper flakes
- ¼ teaspoon ground cumin
- 1 teaspoon smoked paprika
- 4 (4-ounce) grouper fillets, cleaned and patted dry
- 4 tablespoons salted butter, melted
- Juice of 1 lemon

Directions:
1. In a small bowl, stir together the oregano, pepper, salt, cayenne, red pepper flakes, cumin, and paprika. Set aside.
2. Heat your dry skillet over medium-high heat.
3. Brush each fish fillet on both sides with melted butter and carefully coat both sides with the spice mixture.
4. Add the fillets to the hot skillet and cook 2 to 3 minutes per side, until blackened and cooked through.
5. Drizzle the lemon juice over the fish and serve.

239.Veggie-topped Polenta Slices

Servings: 4
Cooking Time: 20 Min
Ingredients:
- 1 tube (1 pound) polenta, cut into 12 slices
- 2 tablespoons olive oil, divided
- 1 medium zucchini, chopped
- 2 shallots, minced
- 2 garlic cloves, minced
- 3 tablespoons reduced-sodium chicken broth
- 1/2 teaspoon pepper
- 1/8 teaspoon salt
- 4 plum tomatoes, seeded and chopped
- 2 tablespoons minced fresh basil or 2 teaspoons dried basil
- 1 tablespoon minced fresh parsley
- 1/2 cup shredded part-skim mozzarella cheese

Directions:
1. In a large nonstick skillet, cook the polenta in 1 tablespoon oil over medium heat for 9-11 minutes on each side or until golden brown.
2. Meanwhile, in another large skillet, saute zucchini in remaining oil until tender. Add shallots and garlic; cook 1 minute longer. Add the broth, pepper and salt. Bring to a boil; cook until liquid is almost evaporated.
3. Stir in the tomatoes, basil and parsley; heat through. Serve with polenta; sprinkle with cheese.

240.Brandy-glazed Carrots

Servings: 12 (3/4 Cup Each)
Cooking Time: 30 Min
Ingredients:
- 3 pounds fresh baby carrots
- 1/2 cup butter, cubed
- 1/2 cup honey
- 1/4 cup brandy
- 1/4 cup minced fresh parsley
- 1/2 teaspoon salt
- 1/4 teaspoon pepper

Directions:
1. In a large skillet, bring 1/2 in. of water to a boil. Add carrots. Cover and cook for 5-9 minutes or until crisp-tender. Drain and set aside.
2. In the same skillet, cook butter and honey over medium heat until butter is melted. Remove from heat; stir in brandy. Bring to a boil; cook until liquid is reduced to about 1/2 cup. Add the carrots, parsley, salt and pepper; heat through.

241.Deep Skillet Pizza

Servings: 2
Cooking Time: 40 Minutes
Ingredients:
- ½ pack (4-oz.) of rolled pizza crust/dough, unbaked
- ¼ cup pizza or tomato sauce
- ½ cup mixed vegetables of your choice, e.g., zucchini, corn, eggplants, peppers
- ¼ cup mozzarella cheese
- 2 tbsp. parmesan cheese
- ½ tsp Italian seasoning
- 1 ½ tbsp. olive oil, divided

Directions:
1. Roast the veggies with half the oil, Italian seasoning, salt, and pepper in the oven at 380F for 12 minutes. Remove from the heat and set aside.
2. Grease the bottom of your skillet with oil and add the dough evenly, with the edges touching the sides of the skillet.
3. Let the pizza dough rest and rise for 5 minutes. Sprinkle with half of the mozzarella cheese, and the pizza sauce, the veggies, and sprinkle with the rest of the mozzarella and parmesan cheese.
4. Bake the pizza in the oven for 25 to 30 minutes.
5. Rest for 10 minutes. Slice and serve.

242.Beef & Sweet Pepper Skillet

Servings: 6
Cooking Time: 30 Min
Ingredients:
- 1 pound lean ground beef (90% lean)
- 2 cups water
- 1 can (14 1/2 ounces) diced tomatoes with mild green chilies, undrained
- 1 tablespoon chili powder
- 2 teaspoons beef stock concentrate
- 1/4 teaspoon salt
- 1/8 teaspoon garlic powder
- 2 cups instant brown rice
- 1 medium sweet red pepper, sliced
- 1 medium green pepper, sliced
- 1 cup (4 ounces) shredded Colby-Monterey Jack cheese

Directions:
1. In a large skillet, cook beef over medium heat 6-8 minutes or until no longer pink, breaking into crumbles; drain.
2. Add water, tomatoes, chili powder, beef stock concentrate, salt and garlic powder; bring to a boil. Stir in the rice and peppers. Reduce heat; simmer, covered, 8-10 minutes or until liquid is absorbed. Remove from the heat; sprinkle with cheese. Let stand, covered, until cheese is melted.

243.Pepper Squash Saute

Servings: 4
Cooking Time: 25 Min
Ingredients:
- 1 small onion, chopped
- 1/3 cup each chopped green, sweet red and yellow pepper
- 1 tablespoon butter

- 1 medium zucchini, chopped
- 1 medium yellow summer squash, chopped
- 1 medium carrot, shredded
- 2 garlic cloves, minced
- 1/2 teaspoon salt
- 1/4 teaspoon pepper

Directions:
1. In a large nonstick skillet, saute onion and peppers in butter for 3-4 minutes. Stir in the zucchini, summer squash and carrot; saute 3-4 minutes or until vegetables are tender.
2. Add garlic; cook 1 minute longer or until tender. Sprinkle with salt and pepper.

244.Garlic Naan

Servings: 6 To 8
Cooking Time: 20 Minutes
Ingredients:
- 2 tablespoons dry active yeast
- 1 tablespoon sugar
- ¼ cup olive oil, plus more for greasing
- ¼ cup warm water
- 5 cups bread flour
- 2 teaspoons baking powder
- 1 cup full-fat plain yogurt
- ½ cup whole milk
- 1 stick salted butter, melted
- 5 garlic cloves, minced
- ¼ cup chopped cilantro
- 1 tablespoon sea salt

Directions:
1. In a large bowl, combine the yeast, sugar, olive oil, and water. Stir well and let it sit for 10 minutes.
2. In another bowl, mix the flour and baking powder.
3. Using a whisk, mix the yogurt and milk into the yeast mixture. Add the flour mixture, a little at a time, mixing first with a wooden spoon and then your hands.
4. Knead with your hands for 2 to 3 minutes, until a soft, smooth dough ball forms.
5. Coat a glass bowl with olive oil. Place the dough ball in the bowl, turn once, and cover with a towel. Allow the dough to rise in a warm spot. The dough should double in size after about 2 hours.
6. Turn the dough out onto a floured surface and punch it down slightly. Divide into 10 equal portions and roll each into an oblong shape. The dough should be ¼" thick.
7. In a small bowl, combine the melted butter and minced garlic. Brush each dough round with the garlic butter.
8. Heat your skillet over medium-high heat.
9. Place a dough round on the hot skillet, butter-side down. Cook for 1 to 2 minutes, until the dough begins to brown. Brush the top side with garlic butter and flip.
10. Cook for an additional 1 to 2 minutes until the bottom side is golden brown. Repeat with the remaining dough.
11. As the naan comes off the skillet, brush it once more with garlic butter and put it in an oven or microwave to keep it warm.
12. Sprinkle with cilantro and salt and serve warm.

245.Nashville Hot Chicken

Servings: 8
Cooking Time: 30 Minutes
Ingredients:

- FOR THE MARINADE
- 2 cups buttermilk
- 1 tablespoon red pepper flakes
- 1 tablespoon cayenne
- 1 tablespoon sea salt
- 1½ teaspoons garlic powder
- 8 to 10 mixed bone-in, skin-on chicken breasts and thighs
- FOR THE BREADING
- 3 cups all-purpose flour, divided
- 1 tablespoon red pepper flakes, divided
- 1 tablespoon cayenne, divided
- 1½ teaspoons garlic powder, divided
- 1 tablespoon sea salt, divided
- 4 eggs
- 2 tablespoons apple cider vinegar
- 2 cups bread crumbs
- ¼ cup yellow, coarse, stone-ground grits
- Peanut oil for frying
- FOR THE SPICY OIL
- 2 tablespoons hot sauce
- 2 tablespoons brown sugar
- 1 tablespoon cayenne
- ½ tablespoon smoked paprika
- ½ tablespoon garlic powder
- 1 teaspoon sea salt

Directions:
1. In a large bowl, mix the buttermilk, red pepper flakes, cayenne, salt, and garlic powder.
2. Add the chicken and turn to coat. Cover and marinate overnight in the refrigerator.
3. Line up three small bowls on your counter. In the first bowl, mix 1½ cups of flour, 1½ teaspoons of red pepper flakes, 1½ teaspoons of cayenne, ¼ teaspoon of garlic powder, and 1½ teaspoons of salt. In the second bowl, whisk together the eggs and vinegar. In the third bowl, whisk together the bread crumbs, grits, and remaining flour, red pepper flakes, cayenne, garlic powder, and salt.
4. In your skillet, heat 1 inch of peanut oil over high heat to 375°F.
5. Working with one piece at a time, dip the chicken into the flour mixture, then the egg mixture, and then the bread crumb mixture.
6. Add the chicken to the hot oil and fry the breasts/white meat for 4 to 5 minutes per side and thighs/dark meat for 6 to 7 minutes per side. Do not discard the frying oil.
7. Transfer to a wire rack to cool slightly.
8. In a heat-proof bowl, mix together the hot sauce, brown sugar, cayenne, paprika, garlic powder, salt, and ½ cup of reserved oil. Whisk well. Brush each piece of chicken with the spicy oil on all sides to coat before serving.

246.Green Chile Corn Bread With Whipped Honey Butter

Servings: 4 To 6
Cooking Time: 25 Minutes
Ingredients:
- For the corn bread
- 1 Anaheim pepper
- 2 cups coarse yellow cornmeal
- 1 teaspoon sea salt
- 1 teaspoon baking powder
- 1 teaspoon baking soda
- 1½ cups buttermilk
- 6 tablespoons (¾ stick) salted butter, melted, divided

- 1 large egg
- For the whipped butter
- 8 tablespoons (1 stick) salted butter, at room temperature
- ¼ cup honey

Directions:
1. To make the corn bread: Adjust the oven rack to the top position and turn the broiler to high.
2. Place the Anaheim pepper into the skillet and put it under the broiler for 2 minutes, until the skin begins to blacken. Remove it from the oven and set it aside to cool. Once cooled, seed and dice the pepper.
3. Using oven mitts, adjust the oven rack back to the middle position. Preheat the oven to 400°F and place the skillet into the oven to preheat.
4. In a large bowl, stir together the cornmeal, salt, baking powder, baking soda, and the diced Anaheim pepper.
5. In a small bowl, whisk the buttermilk, 4 tablespoons of melted butter, and the egg until well combined.
6. Using oven mitts, remove the skillet from the oven and brush it with the remaining 2 tablespoons of melted butter. Pour the batter into the preheated skillet and bake for 20 minutes, or until browned on top.
7. To make the whipped butter: In the bowl with a stand mixer fitted with the whisk attachment, or in a medium bowl and using an electric mixer, whip the butter and honey until light and fluffy. Serve the corn bread warm with the whipped butter.

247.Tuscan Chicken

Servings: 4
Cooking Time: 20 Minutes
Ingredients:
- 1 tablespoon olive oil
- 4 boneless, skinless chicken breasts
- ½ teaspoon sea salt
- ¼ teaspoon freshly ground black pepper
- 3 tablespoons salted butter
- 4 garlic cloves, minced
- 2 shallots, sliced
- 12 cherry tomatoes, halved
- 4 cups fresh spinach
- ¼ cup grated Parmesan cheese
- ½ cup heavy cream
- Cooked rice, for serving
- Juice of 1 lemon

Directions:
1. In your skillet, heat the olive oil over medium heat.
2. Add the chicken and season with the salt and pepper. Cook for 6 to 8 minutes per side, until the chicken has browned and reached an internal temperature of 160°F. Remove from the pan and set aside.
3. Add the butter, garlic, and shallots to the skillet. Cook for 2 to 3 minutes, until the shallots begin to soften. Add the tomatoes and spinach. Cook for an additional 2 to 3 minutes, tossing well to coat the spinach.
4. Add the Parmesan and heavy cream to the pan and stir. Return the chicken to the pan and turn twice to coat it in the sauce. Cook an additional 2 to 3 minutes.
5. Serve on a bed of rice, dividing the sauce between four portions. Top with lemon juice.

248.Veggie Tacos

Servings: 4
Cooking Time: 20 Min
Ingredients:
- 8 taco shells
- 3 cups shredded cabbage
- 1 cup sliced onion

- 1 cup julienned sweet red pepper
- 2 tablespoons canola oil
- 2 teaspoons sugar
- 1 can (15 ounces) black beans, rinsed and drained
- 1 cup salsa
- 1 can (4 ounces) chopped green chilies
- 1 teaspoon chili powder
- 1 teaspoon minced garlic
- 1/4 teaspoon ground cumin
- 1/2 cup shredded cheddar cheese
- 1 medium ripe avocado, peeled and sliced

Directions:
1. Heat taco shells according to package directions. Meanwhile, in a large skillet, saute cabbage, onion and red pepper in oil for 5 minutes or until crisp-tender. Sprinkle with sugar.
2. Stir in the beans, salsa, chilies, chili powder, garlic and cumin. Bring to a boil. Reduce the heat; cover and simmer for 5 minutes or until heated through. Spoon into the taco shells. Garnish with cheese and avocado.

249.Rosemary And Garlic Focaccia

Servings: 4 To 6
Cooking Time: 25 Minutes
Ingredients:
- 1 cup warm water
- 1 tablespoon dry active yeast
- 6 tablespoons olive oil, divided
- 1 teaspoon sea salt, divided
- 2½ cups all-purpose flour
- 3 garlic cloves
- 1 tablespoon coarsely chopped rosemary

Directions:
1. Coat a large bowl with olive oil and set aside.
2. In another large bowl, mix together the water, yeast, 2 tablespoons of olive oil, and ½ teaspoon of salt. Let the mixture sit for 10 minutes.
3. Add the flour, a little at a time, stirring with a wooden spoon.
4. When a rough ball has formed, turn it out onto a floured surface. Knead until the dough is pliable and smooth, 10 to 12 minutes.
5. Transfer the dough to the oiled bowl, turn once, and cover lightly with a towel. Allow the dough to rise in a warm place for 1 hour, until the dough has doubled in size.
6. Punch down the dough. Coat your skillet with 2 tablespoons of olive oil and roll the dough into a 12" round. Place in the skillet and cover with a towel. Allow the dough to rise another 40 to 45 minutes.
7. Heat the oven to 400°F.
8. Use your fingers to dimple the dough. Top with the remaining olive oil, garlic, rosemary, and salt.
9. Bake until the focaccia is a light golden brown, about 25 minutes.
10. Allow to cool slightly before serving.

250.Creole Shrimp & Sausage

Servings: 4
Cooking Time: 30 Min
Ingredients:
- 1/2 cup water
- 1/2 cup chicken broth
- 1 cup quick-cooking bulgur
- 1/2 teaspoon chili powder

- 3/4 teaspoon Creole seasoning, divided
- 1/2 pound smoked sausage, cut into 1/4-inch slices
- 2 teaspoons olive oil, divided
- 1 medium onion, chopped
- 1 medium green pepper, chopped
- 2 garlic cloves, minced
- 1 can (16 ounces) kidney beans, rinsed and drained
- 1 can (14 1/2 ounces) diced tomatoes, undrained
- 1/2 pound uncooked jumbo shrimp, peeled and deveined
- 1/2 teaspoon Worcestershire sauce

Directions:

1.　In a small saucepan, bring water and broth to a boil. Stir in the bulgur, chili powder and 1/4 teaspoon Creole seasoning. Reduce heat; cover and simmer for 15 minutes or until tender.

2.　Meanwhile, in a large skillet, brown sausage in 1 teaspoon oil. Remove and keep warm.

3.　In the same skillet, saute the onion and green pepper in remaining oil until tender. Add garlic; cook 1 minute longer. Stir in the beans, tomatoes, shrimp, Worcestershire sauce, sausage and the remaining Creole seasoning. Cook for 3-5 minutes or until shrimp turn pink. Fluff the bulgur with a fork; serve with sausage mixture.

CPSIA information can be obtained
at www.ICGtesting.com
Printed in the USA
LVHW101438150321
681595LV00006B/79

9 781801 666763